ADVERSE EFFECTS OF HORMONAL CONTRACEPTIVES: MYTH AND REALITY

ADVERSE EFFECTS OF HORMONAL CONTRACEPTIVES: MYTH AND REALITY

ROSA SABATINI
EDITOR

Nova Science Publishers, Inc.
New York

Copyright © 2009 by Nova Science Publishers, Inc.

All rights reserved. No part of this book may be reproduced, stored in a retrieval system or transmitted in any form or by any means: electronic, electrostatic, magnetic, tape, mechanical photocopying, recording or otherwise without the written permission of the Publisher.

For permission to use material from this book please contact us:
Telephone 631-231-7269; Fax 631-231-8175
Web Site: http://www.novapublishers.com

NOTICE TO THE READER

The Publisher has taken reasonable care in the preparation of this book, but makes no expressed or implied warranty of any kind and assumes no responsibility for any errors or omissions. No liability is assumed for incidental or consequential damages in connection with or arising out of information contained in this book. The Publisher shall not be liable for any special, consequential, or exemplary damages resulting, in whole or in part, from the readers' use of, or reliance upon, this material.

Independent verification should be sought for any data, advice or recommendations contained in this book. In addition, no responsibility is assumed by the publisher for any injury and/or damage to persons or property arising from any methods, products, instructions, ideas or otherwise contained in this publication.

This publication is designed to provide accurate and authoritative information with regard to the subject matter covered herein. It is sold with the clear understanding that the Publisher is not engaged in rendering legal or any other professional services. If legal or any other expert assistance is required, the services of a competent person should be sought. FROM A DECLARATION OF PARTICIPANTS JOINTLY ADOPTED BY A COMMITTEE OF THE AMERICAN BAR ASSOCIATION AND A COMMITTEE OF PUBLISHERS.

LIBRARY OF CONGRESS CATALOGING-IN-PUBLICATION DATA

ISBN: 978-1-60692-819-6

Available upon request

Published by Nova Science Publishers, Inc. ✦ New York

Contents

Contents	v
Introduction	vii
Part I, Severe Adverse Effects	1
Rosa Sabatini and Giuseppe Loverro	
Part II, Other Effects	25
Rosa Sabatini	
Part III, Cancer Risks	33
R. Sabatini, P. Trerotoli, R. Cagiano, M. Tartagni and G. Serio	
Part IV, Moderate Adverse Effects	75
Rosa Sabatini	
Part V, Mild Adverse Effects	91
Rosa Sabatini and Raffele Cagiano	
Index	123

INTRODUCTION

Hormonal contraception has been an available method of birth control for over four decades Despite this, women's knowledge often moves between myth and reality, and never has another medical finding aroused over similar controversial opinions. Misperceptions, previous personal experience, suggestion by poor experience from other women and influence of mass media , sometimes contribute to noncompliance or drop-out of the used hormonal contraceptive method because of the user's rational or irrational anxieties (1). In fact,this flash-information may lead to a clearcut relationship between negative suggestion and the incidence of emotional refusal(2). Particularly, the mass media continue to show an ambiguous behaviour enhancing the health risks of COCs use with a generic and uncritical manner or emphasizing the good effects of the hormonal contraceptives without informing about their risks. In addition, the current international influence by pharmaceutical companies on one part of the research can contribute to minimize many adverse outcomes of the sexual steroids and to limit a widespread scientific information .It is known that biological and psychological changes are linked to hormonal contraception,and their adverse effects can play an important role in determining acceptability(3). Actually,hormonal contraceptives (COCs) contain both estrogen and progestin or progestin alone. In 1964, ethinyl estradiol (EE) a better tolerated synthetic estrogen, replaced mestranol and, at the moment, is still used. Oral EE, 200 times more potent than estradiol,exerts its action, primarily dose-dependent, on the estrogen-target organs and tissues (endometrium, mammary epithelium, liver,haemostasis and lipid levels).Furthermore, the estrogen primarily controls the menstrual bleeding. Estrogen and progestin work synergically to inhibit ovulation. The androgenic action of progestins, reflected in reduction of HDL cholesterol, is an important factor in occurrence of arterial accidents(4). In the early 1980s,the third generation oral contraceptives were developed in an attempt to decrease the risk of cardiovascular disease (CVD) and to decrease androgenic side-effects such as weight gain,acne and adverse changes in metabolism of lipoproteins. Although the major disadvantage of third generation COCs, according with the majority of authors, is the increased risk of vascular effects (5,6).Anyway, the third-generation 19-nortestosterone derivatives(gestodene, desogestrel, norgestimate), allowed the reduction of the COCs steroid doses.In the last decade, with the aim to decrease the adverse effects- COCs related and to enhance the user's compliance, besides the dose reduction, other approaches have been performed such as the improvement in previous methods, the development of new steroids and the characterization of new schedules of administration. Currently, new available options of non-daily hormonal contraception, utilizing classic or alternative routes of administration, are present on the market .Today the long-acting contraceptives constitute an important option in the family planning services of several countries. We remember the long-lasting action(5 years) levonorgestrel-releasing intrauterine device(IUD)(20μg/day), the monthly injectable Lunelle (25 mg medroxyprogesterone cypionate + 5 mg estradiol),the monthly intravaginal ring containing 15μg ethinylestradiol and 120 μg etonogestrel, the weekly transdermal patch releasing 20 μg ethinylestradiol and 150 μg norelgestromin(active metabolite of norgestimate) over 24 hours, the subdermal implant (Implanon) containing 68 mg of etonogestrel. In addition,it is important to remember the new generation of oral antiandrogenic progestins as drospirenone and clormadinone acetate-containing COCs. In the mean time , extended or continuous regimens were experienced introducing the new idea of contraception without menstruation.These new means of administration obtained legitimacy through their use in treating endometriosis, dysmenorrhea,and menstrual-symptoms ; however, some women without problems likewise, prefer to avoid their periods. Eventual long-time adverse effects related to these new regimens are hitherto unknown. From the experience of the post-menopausal women, long-term taking hormonal replacement therapy, a possible deleterious effect time-related might be hypothesized(7). Therefore until now, no contraceptive exists without some adverse effect. Besides, little is known about the relationship between the safety of hormonal contraceptives and the risk of breast cancer among BRCA 1 / 2 mutation carriers (8,9). Currently, the large variety of the hormonal contraceptive preparations, the different doses and the different formulations, the different routes of administration, and the right of all women to avoid an unwilling pregnancy, created a complex scenario. Moreover, many teenagers are sexually active at earlier ages than in the past, before they are cognitively able to develop a responsible sexual behavior(10). Therefore, considering the frequency of their sexual intercourses and the short lasting of sexual partnerships, effective contraceptive counselling for adolescent should be an absolute necessity. Nevertheless, the adherence to COCs is often poor; concerns about side-effects, especially those affecting the menstrual cycle and the body weight, are often given as reason for discontinuation. Consequently, unwilling pregnancies in adolescents remain a widespread social problem in all developed countries; in fact, five million abortions carried out yearly worldwide concern girls aged 15-19(11). Then, it is mandatory to provide for a safe method of birth control in this age-group and to avoid the method discontinuation. However, the contraception management of these young women may encounter serious problems among those unaware carriers of the "factor V Leiden mutation" or with other kind of diseases, especially affecting hemostatic system (12,13,14).

Furthermore, there is an emerging evidence for requiring contraception in women aged 40 and older in which the occurrence of unintended pregnancy represents a significant problem. Adverse effects in healthy women taking hormonal contraceptives, are never accepted and can lead to poor compliance. In addition, clinical researches reported a statistically significant correlation between undesirable side-effects and impairment of sexual function resulting in a very high considerable aspect in this age-group. Although fertility naturally declines with advancing age, women in their forties wish to continue to be sexually active long beyond their desire for childbearing. Then contraception becomes a great consideration during the last reproductive years. Current researches indicated the safety of extending the use of combined hormonal contraceptives (COCs) to healthy women beyond the age of 40 and up to menopause without the need for replacement (15). Women should still use contraception until 1 year after the last menstrual period because irregular ovulation may occur. Since well-designed studies proved an increased risk of thromboembolism with aging and with estrogen dose,it is wise to prescribe the lowest available dose of ethinylestradiol(EE) in the COCs for adequately counselled couples(16).Furthermore, women's age, obesity and family history of hypertension were associated with an increase of blood pressure and this event resulted independent of the contraceptive used.(17).Besides, the low affinity to androgen receptors of some progestins could influence the endogenous androgen environment in the direction of hypoandrogenism(3,18). A lot of studies suggest that the androgens play an important role in modulating the female sexual arousal.In addition, beginning in their 30s, women slowly lose circulating testosterone and significant associations between low sexual responsiveness and age are reported.It is necessary to make an accurate selection of the middle aged women considering the high risk of adverse effects of this age-group. Generally, disturbances –COC related, are mild or moderate in level ; rarely,severe and only sporadic fatal cases are reported. Whatever the case, severe adverse effects exist; perhaps they are very rare, but it might be that other cases were underestimated or ignored(19,20,21).Therefore,also mild or moderate adverse effects of COCs may impact the woman's quality of life. Particularly,considering the modern lifestyle, more importance is devoted to loss of desire caused by some COCs and their capability to heavily influence the relational and intimate life (18). Besides, even small increases in frequency of adverse effects in COCs -users have a general critical health impact because of their widespread use, which is currently expanding to potential risk groups (22). In fact, women transplanted, depressed,suffering cardiovascular diseases, diabetes, neoplasms , thrombophilic syndromes or rare diseases and/or smokers, today seek contraception(23). Therapy selection should be individualized and based on the patient's specific needs and global related health risks. In addition, for the management of these cases and the individual risk evaluation, specific knowledge is necessary about the particular pathologic entity and the possible contraceptive action.In fact, the superficial evaluation can lead to refuse a safe contraceptive method when suitable, or to prescribe a hormonal contraceptive when hazardous. These circumstances,at the worst, could be object of serious legal proceedings. Surveillance of the user's health and follow-up are needed. Consequently, an accurate contraceptive counselling,a good experience in this field and an optimal knowledge of each contraceptive method, together with its potential adverse effects, are mandatory for a modern contraceptive strategy.

REFERENCES

[1] Mall-Haefeli, M. (1980). Internal medecine problems regarding contraception. Part 1. *Schweiz Med.Wochenschr*, 110(36), 1314-9.
[2] Grady, W.R.,Billy, J.O., Klepinger, D.H. (2002).Contraceptive method switching in the United States. *Perspect.Sex Reprod.Health*, 34(3),135-45.
[3] Sabatini, R.,Cagiano, R. (2006).Comparison profiles of cycle control,side-effects and sexual satisfaction of three hormonal contraceptives.*Contraception*, 74,220-223
[4] Belaisch, J., Eliakim, V. (1993). Third generation progestagens. Contracept. Fertil. *Sex* (Paris), 21(4), 287-93.
[5] Gerstman, B.B., Piper, J.M., Tomita, D.K., Ferguson, W.J., Stadel, B.V., Lundin, E.E. (1991). Oral contraceptive estrogen dose and the risk of deep venous thromboembolic disease. *Am.J. Epidemiol*, 133, 32-37.

[6] Kemmeren, J.M., Algra, A.,Grobbee, D.E. (2001). Third generation oral contraceptives and risk of venous thrombosis:meta-analysis. *Br.Med.J*, 323,131-134.
[7] Geist, R., Beyth, Y. Extended cycle oral contraceptives.Harefuah, 2007;146(10):781-4,813.
[8] Haile, R.W.,Thoma, D.C., McGuire, V., Felberg, A., John, E.M., Milne, R.L., Hopper, J.L. et al. (2006). BRCA1 and BRCA2 mutation carriers,oral contraceptives use,and breast cancer before age 50. Cancer Epidemiol.*Biomarker Prev*, 15(10),1863-70.
[9] Brohet, R.M.,Goldgar, D.E., Easton, D.F., Antoniou, A.C., Andrieu, N., Chang-Claude, J. et al. (2007).Oral contraceptives and breast cancer in the international BRCA 1 / 2 carrier cohort study:a report from EMBRACE,GENEPSO,GEO-HEBON and the IBCCS Collaborating Group. *J.Clin.Oncol*, 25(25),3831-6.
[10] Sabatini, R.,Orsini, G.,Cagiano, R., Loverro, G. (2007). Noncontraceptive benefits of two combined oral contraceptives with antiandrogenic properties among adolescents.*Contraception*, 76, 342-347.
[11] Garden, A.S. (2003). *Teenage pregnancy*. In Amy JJ ed,.Paediatric and adolescent gynaecology.Amsterdam.Elsevier, 263-70.
[12] Bloemenkamp, K.W., Rosendaal, F.R., Helmerhorst, F.M., Buller, H.R.,Vandenbroucke, J.P. (1995). Enhancement by factor V Leiden mutation of risk of deep –vein thrombosis associated with oral contraceptives containing a third-generation progestagens.*Lancet*, 346,1593-6.
[13] Comp, P.C., Rsmonm C,T. (1984). Recurrent venous thromboembolism in patients with a partial deficiency of protein S. *N. Engl.J.Med*, 311,1525-1528).
[14] Schwartz, S.M.,Siscovick, D.S., Longstreth, W.T., Psaty, B.M., Beverly, R.K., Raghunathan, T.E., Lin, D. (1997). Use of Low –Dose Oral Contraceptives and Stroke in Young Women. *Annals Int.Med*, Vol.127 Issue 8(part 1), 596-603.
[15] Shaaban, M.M. (1996).The perimenopause and contraception.*Maturitas*, 23(2), 181-92
[16] Speroff, L., Sulak, P.J. (1995).Contraception in the later reproductive years :a valid aspect of preventive health care. *Dialogues Contracept*, 4(5), 1-4.
[17] Shen, Q., Lin, D., Jiang, X., Li, H., Zhang, Z. (1994). Blood pressure changes and hormonal contraceptives.*Contraception*, 50(2), 131-41.
[18] Dennerstein, L., Duldey, E.C., Hopper, J.C., Burger, H. (1997). Sexuality,hormones and the menopausal transition.*Maturitas*, 26, 83-93.

[19] Petitti, D.B., Sidney, S.,Quesenberry, C.P. (1998). Oral contraceptive useand myocardial infarction. *Contraception*, 57, 143-155.
[20] Parkin, L., Skegg, D.C.,Wilson, M.et al. (2000).Oral contraceptives and fatal pulmonary embolism. *Lancet*, 355, 2133-34,
[21] Jick, H., Jick, S.S.,Gurewich, V., Myers, M.W., Vasilakis, C. (1995). Risk of idiopathic cardiovascular death and nonfatal venous thromboembolism in women using oral contraceptives with differing progestagen components.*Lancet*, 346, 1589-93.
[22] Petersen, K.R. (2002).Pharmacodynamic effects of oral contraceptives steroid on biochemical markers for arterial thrombosis.Studies in non-diabetic women and in women with insulin-dependent diabetes mellitus. *Dan.Med. Bull*, 49(1), 43-60).
[23] Sondheimer S.J. (1991).Update on the methabolic effects of steroidal contraceptives. Endocrinol. *Metab. Clin. North Am*, 20(4), 911-23

In: Adverse Effects of Hormonal Contraceptives
Editor: R. Sabatini

ISBN: 978-1-60692-819-6
© 2009 Nova Science Publishers, Inc.

PART I, SEVERE ADVERSE EFFECTS

Rosa Sabatini and Giuseppe Loverro
Dept.Obstetrics and Gynecology,
General Hospital Policlinico-University of Bari, Italy

Cardiovascular Effects

The first report about a case of pulmonary embolism as adverse effect of contraception occurred in 1961(1).

MYOCARDIAL INFARCTION

In the last years,the incidence of myocardial infarction(MI)was estimated of 2 to5 fold for hormonal contraceptive (HC)-users compared with nonusers(2,3).The risk results dose-related ,and increased also for women using low-dose pill. Coagulation factors, especially factors VII and fibrinogen, have been established as important cardiovascular risk factors in men. Some studies have shown the levels of factors VII and fibrinogen to be elevated in HC users. These procoagulant alterations are also observed in women receiving estrogen substitution, but unlike HC users, such women appear to be protected by age-related increases in the level of antitrombin III(4,5). Smoking is an important influence-factor on the fibrinogen level, which probably explains part of the increased risk of MI among HC users.Both ,smoking and hypertension substantially increase the risk among HC users and some data suggest an increased risk among women with diabetes, hypercholesterolaemia or a history of pre-eclampsia or hypertension-pregnancy related. The role of the different types of progestagens used in HCs is still controversial (6,7,8). Clinical trials on myocardial infarction have found inconsistent results, possibly because of differences in the prevalence of risk factors, particularly smoking and elevated blood pressure, in the populations studied. In the absence of a history of smoking and other conventional risk factors, current users of modern COCs probably do not have an increased risk of myocardial infarction. Neither are former users at risk(9). Evidence for important differences in the risk of myocardial infarction between formulations is weak and contradictory. However, a study carried out on 217 women with a first myocardial infarction before the age of 50 years, and 763 healthy control women showed that the risk is substantially elevated among women with various inherited clotting factor defects(10). The overall odds ratio for myocardial infarction, in the presence of a coagulation defect is 1.1. The combination of a prothrombotic mutation and current smoking, increases the risk of myocardial infarction 12- fold compared with non-smokers, without a coagulation defect.Among women who smoke cigarettes, factor V Leiden presence versus absence increases the risk by 2.0,and prothrombin 20210A mutation presence versus absence has an odds ratio of 1.0(11).Nevertheless, some studies reported that the risk of myocardial infarction does not appear to depend on coagulation abnormalities or the type of oral contraceptive. However, the risk is highest in the first year of use and increases in women with a previous venous thrombosis and with age.In the past years was demonstrated, on 219 death from myocardial infarction,that the frequency of use of combined oral contraceptives (COCs), during the month before death was significantly greater in the group with infarction than in the control group and the average duration of use was longer(12) The lowering of the estrogen dose in COCs from 50 mcg to 20-30 mcg, in the last decade, clearly does not reduce the risk of myocardial infarction;although current opinions are conflicting(13,14).The effects in COC users with other risk factors for venous thrombosis tend to be less pronounced and more inconsistent. A number of studies have found higher relative risks among current users of low estrogen dose COCs containing desogestrel or gestodene, than among users of similar products containing levonorgestrel (14). A number of explanations, in terms of bias or confounding, have been proposed for these clinically small differences.At best, empirical evidence for these explanations is weak. A transnational study carried out on 182 women aged 18-44 with myocardial infarction(MI) compared with 635 women without MI reported overall odds ratio for MI for second generation COC versus no current users of 2.35 and 0.82 for third generation. A direct comparison of third generation users with second generation users yielded an OR of 0.28(OR=odds ratio). Among users of third generation combined oral contraceptive(COC), the OR for current smokers was 3.75, and among users of second generation it was 9.50.(13).In conclusion ,myocardial infarction in women taking combined hormonal contraceptives remains rare; in fact,it has been estimated that the population attributable risk is less than three events in one million women years(3).A logical hypothesis to explain the development of myocardial infarction would be an interaction between the hypercoagulability induced by COCs and the risk factors,known or unknown,in the users(15). It is interesting to remember that antibodies to synthetic steroids (ethinylestradiol and progesterone) and circulating immune complexes were found in the serum of 30% of HC users and their titres are significantly higher in 90% of women who develop vascular thrombosis unrelated to atherosclerosis(16,17).In the last years, sporadic cases of myocardial infarction associated with hormonal contraceptive have been reported(17,18,19).Women can minimize, and possibly eliminate entirely, their arterial risks by not smoking and by having their blood pressure checked before using a COC in order to avoid its use if elevated blood pressure is discovered. The users may decrease their venous thromboembolic risk by their choice of COC preparation although the effects will be modest. Thus, reducing the hormone dosage of COCs and performing better screening of patients are needed to further reduce the frequency of cardiovascular complications.

STROKE

Most users of hormonal contraceptives (HCs) have a low background incidence of major cardiovascular diseases. In fact,current users of low estrogen dose – HC s have a small increased risk of ischaemic stroke, although most of the risk occurs in women with other risk factors, notably hypertension, age,smoking, and a history of migraine(20,21,22). Particularly ,the risk of ischaemic stroke among current users with a history of hypertension was evaluated 10.7(odds ratio)(23). Similarly, the use of HC increases the risk of haemorrhagic stroke in women aged over 35 years (odds ratio greater than 2)and when they have a history of hypertension, this risk is 10-15 fold compared with women who did not use COC s and did not have a history of hypertension(24). Odds ratio among current users who are also current cigarette smokers was greater than 3. Past users of HCs do not seem to have an increased risk of stroke. The risks are similar for subarachnoid and intracerebral haemorrhage.(25). After the introduction of low-dose oral contraceptives,a decline in cerebral thromboembolism among young women has been reported

(26). However, cerebrovascular occlusion in young women may be caused by hormonal contraceptive use when unsuspected free protein S or protein C deficiency, coagulation factor XIII gene variation or inherited thrombophilia exist(27,28, 29,30).The role of inherited prothrombotic conditions as factor V Leiden, and prothrombin mutation in the pathogenesis of ischemic stroke is not well established; although it seems that carriers of the factor V Leiden mutation might have a 11.2 fold higher risk of ischemic stroke than women without either risk factor(31,32) .A prospective cohort study on 44,408 women on low-dose oral contraceptives and 75,230 with an intrauterine device(IUD) followed during three years, reported a higher incidence of haemorrhagic stroke than ischemic stroke(34.74 versus 11.25 per 100,000 woman years)for HC users .The relative risk(RR) of incidence of haemorrhagic stroke was 2.72 times compared with that in the IUD users. Furthermore, the RR of current users of HC was 4.20 and still reached 2.17 among past users after they stopped taking HC for more than 10 years(33).While,other studies had found no statistically significant increase in the risk of stroke among HC past users without other risk factors.In fact, for past users compared with never users the odds ratio was 0.59(34) Current users of low-dose oral contraceptives had a risk for stroke similar to that of women who have never used these medications and the results did not differ appreciably between hemorrhagic stroke and ischaemic stroke. Although other studies reported that the incidence of total stroke among 18-44 –year-old was 11.3 per 100,000 women-years, and the rate of haemorrhagic stroke was higher than the rate of ischemic stroke (6.4 per 100.000 women-year compared with 4.3 per 100.000 women-year). Compared with women who had never used com bined oral contraceptives(COCs),current users of low-dose COCs had estimated odds tatio of 0.93 for hemorrhagic stroke and 0.89 for ischemic stroke(35,36,37).There is insufficient information to determine whether major differences in the risk of ischaemic stroke exist between different formulations. Data examining the risk of haemorrhagic stroke in current COC users with other risk factors are very sparse, as are those relating to the haemorrhagic stroke risk associated with particular COCs. Literature data are scarce and sometimes showed methodological limitations.There is a discrepancy between the different studies.It is important to remember that we define stroke as the rapid onset of loss of cerebral function that lasted at least 24 hours and could not be ascribed to subdural hematoma or to other diseases: neurologic, neoplastic,infection,seizure or multiple sclerosis. The stroke may be venous or arterial in origin and the second may be hemorragic , ischemic or provoked by other cause as the arterial dissection.The aneurysmal bleeding was defined as a haemorrhagic stroke. The role of hormonal contraceptives (HCs)as a risk factor for cerebrovascular pathology is still discussed.Various prospective and retrospective studies to establish the causal or casual relationship between HC use and stroke are necessary (38). A recent study found that women using HCs had a relative risk for cerebrovascular accidents of 1.5. The risk was increased at higher doses and for some specific progestins. No evidence supports a relationship between atherogenic disease and use of COCs. Former users of HCs do not have an increased risk of ischaemic stroke(38). In addition , it is important to evaluate the relationship between migraine and stroke considering the high prevalence of migraine in young women.(39). It is reported that a significant association between migraine with aura and juvenile stroke in women exist with the odds ratio of 2.11 in women aged under 46 years and 3.26 under the age of 35(40,41). Migraine with visual aura was associated with an increased risk of stroke; particularly , those who smoke and with other medical conditions associated, when take oral contraceptives markedly increase the risk(40, 41).There is insufficient information to determine whether major differences in the risk of ischaemic stroke exist between products. Current users appear to have a modestly elevated risk of haemorrhagic stroke, mainly in women older than 35 years; former users do not. Cases of transitory ischemic attacks in women with migraine have been reported,also with progesterone-only preparation(42)In most cases of myocardial infarction or stroke, one or more risk factors were identified (39,43). Cerebral vein and sinus thrombosis may occur in COC users affected by congenital thrombophilia, especially if prothrombotic conditions like hyperhomocysteinemia, nephrotic syndrome ,or if unknown, dural arteriovenous malformations are present(19). Fortunately, these findings are reported only in sporadic cases. It is essential to provide the preventive diagnosis with the aim to avoid a probable high risk for the woman; therefore, recent research has shown the influence of the type of progestin. Despite the limited data,it seems that progestin-only-contraceptive does not increase the risk of heart attack and stroke.Until now,no sufficient Literature data exist about combined hormonal contraceptives delivered by a different route (transdermal patch, vaginal ring , subdermal implant).Instead, a cohort study reported no stroke relief among 49,048 women-years of transdermal contraceptive system exposure, and 10 among norgestimate-containing oral contraceptive users (44).In conclusion, current available studies indicate that there is no significant increase in the risk of ischaemic stroke or acute myocardial infarction associated with the use of low-dose estrogen COCs in women properly screened before use, and who have no pre-existing cardiovascular risk factors.

ARTERIAL ACCIDENTS

Among women taking combined hormonal contraceptives(COCs), arterial accidents rarely occur, and isolated cases are reported also, in women taking only-progestin preparations (POP). In the meantime, the lowering of the ethinylestradiol dose of hormonal contraceptives (HCs), accompanied by a steady decline in venous accidents, clearly did not reduce the risk of arterial accidents(31). Furthermore, arterial thrombosis seems to be unrelated to the duration of use or past use of COCs(2,26). Several studies have indicated that smoking and age with hypertension ,diabetes and, hypercholesterolemia are most important risk factors as well as thrombophilia(6,37,39,43,45). The mortality from arterial diseases is 3.5 times higher than the number of deaths from venous diseases in women under 30 years taking COC s and 8.5 times higher in those 30-44 years old.Moreover,COCs with second generation of progestagens seem to confer a smaller increase in the risk of venous diseases and a higher risk of arterial complications,compared with COCs containing third generation progestagens(46,47). In addition, epidemiologic studies suggest that arterial disease risk in young women decreases within 5-10 years of smoking cessation(48).Nevertheless, it is believed that COC use, per se, does not cause arterial disease, it can synergize with subclinical endothelial damage to promote arterial occlusion. The prothrombotic effect of the hormonal contraceptive estrogen intervenes in a cycle of endothelial damage and repair which would otherwise remain clinically silent ,or would ultimately progress because of presence of smoking, hypertension or other factors, to atherosclerosis (47,48). Therefore, the risk of arterial diseases does not seem to increase in healthy non smoker women under 35 years (49). However, a study performed on 152 women with peripheral arterial disease (PAD) and 925 control women(age 18-49 years) affirmed that all types of COC s were associated with an increase of PAD (50). The same results were obtained from a rigorous meta-analysis of the Literature from 1980 to 2002(33).The effects of COCs on the haemostasis and inflammation variables,resulting in an increased thrombosis risk,show large differences in the women's response and the polymorphism in the estrogen receptor-1 (ER1) gene may explain part of this inter-individual response.However,a recent research evidenced that the haplotype ER-1, does not have a strong effect on the estrogen-induced changes in haemostasis and inflammation risk markers for arterial and venous thrombosis. In fact ,in this study no significant link between the different doses of ethinylestradiol and the effect was found (51).In the Literature, some cases of isolated or multiple artery occlusions in young women who smoke and who take oral contraceptives have been reported(47,52,53).Scarce data are available on involvement of progestins in the coagulation patho-mechanisms. However, likely the vascular effects of progestins are mediated through progestin receptors as well as through down-regulation of estradiol receptors [54,55]. Estrogen and progestin receptors are localized in endothelial and smooth muscle cells of the vessel wall, but there are differences in the response of vein and arteries to sex-steroids. In the arteries, the progestin may inhibit the endothelium-dependent vasodilatator action of estrogens; while, in the veins progestin may increase the capacitance resulting in a decreased blood flow. Modification in hemostasis parameters seems to depend on the type and dose of progestogen, the presence of estrogen compound and the duration of use. The risk of combined formulation could be a consequence of vascular action of progestins. In fact, it seems that some progestins may up-regulate thrombin receptor expression, while other progestins did not (56,57).Definitive conclusions about the significance of these findings have not yet been achieved. In this light, the prudent choice of hormonal regimen could be recommended. Using progestins with minimal vascular toxicity may lead to the safety of estrogen-progestin preparations for pre-menopausal women also with Hereditary Hemorrhagic Telangiectasia(HHT). In fact, COC use seems to be a promising alternative to usual treatment of nosebleeds, also as a first –line option in women HHT- affected. In the meantime, this management avoids the risk of pregnancy(58). Further studies are required to establish the role of progestins on haemostasis(59). Generally ,there was no evidence of a significantly increased risk of arterial wall disease in healthy non smoker users under 35 years. No differences between second and third generation oral contraceptives on the risk of arterial wall disease were found. In most cases of myocardial infarction or stroke, one or more risk factors were identified. Two of the most relevant risk factors are smoking and the absence of blood pressure control without forgetting the thrombophilic syndromes,particularly when unrecognized(60).When COC s are prescribed to women with known risk factors for arterial thrombotic disease such as smoking,diabetes, hypertension, migraine with aura, family disposition of acute myocardial infarction or thrombotic stroke, a low-dose pill with a third generation progestins may have an advantage, particularly over 30 years.

VENOUS THROMBOEMBOLISM

Venous thromboembolism(VTE)is a common disorder,and oral contraceptives(OC) are well-known risk factors associated with venous thromboembolism(VTE)(2,15,44,49)The individual risk of VTE varies as a result of a complex interaction between congenital and transient or permanent acquired risk factors. Risk factors can be either intrinsic as age, overweight, previous VTE,thrombophilia or related to surgical procedures, and/ or to medical disorders such as neoplastic diseases(61,62).Inherited thrombophilia is a very important risk factor of venous thromboembolism(VTE)however, there are only few studies on the risk of VTE in women with inherited thrombophilia who use oral contraceptives(63,64).Retrospective family cohort studies revealed the absolute risk of venous thromboembolism in women with single or multiple thrombophilic defects taking hormonal contraceptives(64,65,66).Because of the high prevalence of the carriers of the G20E10A mutation of the prothrombin gene(PT20210A)(6.5%)and the carriers of the factor V Leiden mutation (FVL) (2%) (a hereditary disorder in which activated factor V is inactivated by activated protein C)in the Spanish population, a retrospective family cohort study of 325 women, belonging to 97 families with inherited thrombophilia, was performed to determine the risk of VTE associated with hormonal contraceptives(HCs) intake.The results of this study showed for carriers of the PT20210A mutation, the risk of VTE in HC users was 3-fold higher than that in non-carriers.Carriers of FVL(FactorV Leiden)mutation taking HCs showed an OR of 1.4,indicating a tendency to increase the risk of VTE(67).Genetic screening for these mutations should be considered in potential OC users belonging to families with thrombophilia (68).Women with hereditary deficiencies of protein S, protein C or antithrombin are at high risk of VTE when taking hormonal contraceptives, particularly if other thrombophilic defects are present (69,70,71). Generally, they have VTE at a younger age, and sometimes this event may be dramatic but the overall risk is not increased by HCs (72,73,74,75).In addition, rare cases of thromboembolism in young women caused from the increase of coagulation factor VIII were reported(76,77). A retrospective study compared the venous impact of chlormadinone acetate, at antigonadotropic doses, versus no hormonal treatment in 204 women at high risk of venous thromboembolism. During follow-up (mean of 33 months) nine episodes of VTE were observed: three in women receiving CMA and six in untreated women. Using the Cox model to adjust for confounding variables such as age, thrombophilia and body mass index, the relative risk of VTE associated with the use of CMA was not significant [relative risk:RR 0.8 (78).Therefore, which is the risk of VTE in normal women taking hormonal contraceptives? The risk of venous thromboembolism seems primarily dependent on the dose of ethinylestradiol; although the potential contribution of the new progestins in reducing vascular risks is of great importance (2,15,44,49). Unfortunately, the major disadvantage of third generation HCs ,according to most authors, is the increased risk of vascular effects. (22,55,79). These events seem more pronounced during the first year of use(5,48). In 1995, an important study reported that desogestrel and gestodene could increase the risk of venous thromboembolism and showed an antagonist effect of LNG on the EE-induced rise of factor VII activity and on the EE-induced reduction of total and free protein S(26,36,42). In addition, the effects of a combined oral contraceptive containing 20mcg EE and 75mcg gestodene(GSD)on hemostatic parameters were investigated. Results showed no significant changes in fibrinogen,protein C,AT III or D-dimer during COC use.While the increase in platelet count, decrease in protein S level, prothrombin activity and activated partial thromboplastin time, and the prolongation of thrombin time were significant(80).Furthermore,the thrombotic risk with the use of particular third-generation oral contraceptives was elevated among carriers of the factor V Leiden mutation.This disorder is a common risk factor for venous thrombosis,which is associated with a 3 to 7-fold increased risk in heterozygous individuals (61,62, 81,82).A plausible logical mechanism for the thrombotic effects of second and third-generation oral contraceptives is still lacking.Rosing reported that oral contraceptive use leads to acquired activated protein C(APC)resistance and women using third-generation HCs are more resistant to the anticoagulant action of APC than users of second-generation HCs(83,84).The difference could be explained by differential effects of progestagens on plasma sensitivity to activated protein C (APC). A study assessed the effect of APC on endogenous thrombin potential (ETP) in the plasma of healthy women using either, combined HC or progestagen-only OC,and in non-users.Carriers of factor V Leiden were excluded. Compared with non-users, there was no significant change in APC resistance in women using progestagen-only HC(chlormadinone acetate). Women who used combined HC were less sensitive to APC than non-users ($P < 0.001$) and the difference was significantly more pronounced in women using third-generation HC than in those who used second-generation OC containing levonorgestrel($P < 0.05$).Compared with HC containing levonorgestrel, the use of norethisterone-containing HC was associated with an increased resistance to APC ($P < 0.05$). Women who used cyproterone-containing HC (n = 10) were less sensitive to APC than those using third-generation HC ($P < 0.05$) or second-generation HC containing levonorgestrel ($P < 0.05$) (78,85). Few data are available on involvement of progestins in the coagulation patho-mechanisms. It is, therefore,likely that the vascular effects of progestins are mediated through progestin receptors as well as through down-regulation of estradiol receptors [54,56,59]. Estrogen and progestin receptors are localized in endothelial and smooth muscle cells of the vessel wall, but there are differences in the response of vein and arteries to sex-steroids(49). In fact, in the veins progestins may increase the capacitance resulting in a decrease blood flow[

48,49]. Modification in hemostasis parameters seems to depend to type and dose of progestogen, the presence of estrogen compound and the duration of use[57,85,86]. The risk of combined formulation could be a consequence of vascular action of progestins. In fact, it seems that some progestins may up-regulate thrombin receptor expression while, other progestins did not.[59]. Definitive conclusions about the significance of these findings have not yet achieved. In this light, the prudent choice of hormonal regimen could be recommended.

Using progestins with minimal vascular toxicity may lead to relative safety of estrogen-progestin preparations for pre-menopausal women, also HHT-affected [58]. Desogestrel is less androgenic than previous generations of synthetic progestins.Consequently, when the dose of EE in HC was reduced, the potency of progestagens was increased.Moreover, progestagens with no or reduced androgenic activity were preferred for use in HC with respect to lipid and carbohydrate metabolism(87) .A beneficial effect of these progestins on the coagulation factors is less apparent. It has been suggested that with a reduced androgenic effect of the progestins,the activity of ethinylestradiol is more sensible ,since the estrogens are the source of disturbance in coagulation factors.The third generation of progestins does not appear to represent an advance in reducing arterial accidents ,whereas the reduction from 50 to 30 mcg of ethinylestradiol did in reducing venous pathology. Moreover, the crude rate of VTE per 10.000 woman years was 4.10 in current users : 3.10 in users of second- generation HCs,and 4.96 in users of third- generation HCs.Among users of third generation progestagens,the risk of VTE was higher in users of desogestrel(DSG) with 20 mcg EE than in users of gestodene or desogestrel with 30 mcg EE .The odds-ratio for VTE was estimated 3.49 in the first case and 1.18 for the others.(86,87).The risk of VTE in users of desogestrel-containing HCs is significantly elevated compared to that of LNG –containing HCs. While,the risk of VTE in users of norgestimate-containing HCs was similar to that of users of LNG-containing HCs. (88,89). Unexpected idiopathic cardiovascular death rates among 303.470 women who were current HCs, users were 4.3/100.000 for LNG,1.5/100.000 for desogestrel(DSG) and 4.8/100.000 for gestodene. When compared with LNG the relative risk adjusted for age and calendar period was 0.4 for DSG and 1.4 for gestodene HCs(86,87).The studies carried out on women with and without family history of thrombosis and /or carrier of the factor V Leiden mutation treated with DSG-containing HCs reported the same risk of deep –vein-thrombosis (DVT).This risk resulted higher of 2.2-fold when compared with LNG-containing HCs with the same amount of EE and it was highest in the youngest age categories(82,90,91,92). The increased fibrinolytic activity during HCs use appears to be induced by the estrogen component and may be the result of an enhanced down-regulation of fibrinolysis (26,51,82,90)

Compared to second generation,the use of third generation oral contraceptives has been associated with an increased risk of venous thrombosis ,especially in women with the factor V Leiden mutation(87,91).These HCs induce a decrease in factor V, whereas the levels of all other coagulant factors increased.Several studies demonstrate that many progestins markedly potentiate the vascular procoagulant effects of thrombin by increasing the availability of membrane thrombin receptors in the smooth muscle and this effect seems linked to their glucocorticoid-like-activity(59) .When the women used POP(progestin-only pill) ,a differential effect from DSG and LNG was only found for factor IX. While, in women at high risk of VTE(previous documented history of deep vein thrombosis or pulmonary embolism, carriers of a congenital or acquired thrombophilia or history of a severe/fatal venous thrombosis in a first-degree family member)chlormadinone acetare(17α hydroxyprogesterone derivative)only, used at antigonadotropic doses during 18-20 cycles ,was not associated with a significant increase in the risk of VTE(78). In carriers of the factor V Leiden mutation, DSG-containing oral contraceptives induce more pronounced changes in factor V and in factor VII compared with LNG. Comparing DSG and LNG only,exclusively for factor V a differential effect was found. It appears that DSG-containing oral contraceptives have a more pronounced effect on the coagulation system than LNG-containing oral contraceptives which may explained by a less effective compensation of the thrombotic effect of ethinylestradiol by desogestrel (51,61,87,91,92) When compared to COCs containing LNG or norethisterone, these containing desogestrel or gestodene present a two-fold greater risk of VTE.For COCs containing cyproterone acetate,the risk is four-fold greater,while there are no or insufficient data for those containing norgestimate,chlormadinone acetate or drospirenone(86,88,91, 92).Deep venous thrombosis with pulmonary embolus is a rare complication of oral contraceptives, which generally occurs in adult women and becomes more common with increasing age(87,90). Nevertheless, these complication are believed to be less common with low-dose oral contraceptives than with high doses, a case of thromboembolism with a life-threatening pulmonary embolism in an adolescent on low dose triphasic oral contraceptives has been reported(73).In the development of these thrombotic events, secondary hypercoagulable states may have an important relief. However, these are complex clinical conditions associated with an increased risk of thrombosis in which the exact patho physiology is still poorly understood(94).With regard to the contraceptive patch,the available data suggest that the risk of VTE is similar to that observed with COCs. In the last years ,several studies found a relatively moderate risk of non fatal venous thromboembolism in the contraceptive patch(ethinylestradiol/ norelgestromin) users. Despite this, the contraceptive patch may be an appropriate option for many women. Nevertheless, some studies reported that the increase in activated protein resistance is greater with the patch than with either triphasic and monophasic COCs.(95) .There are no sufficient data concerning vaginal rings.

In conclusion , epidemiological studies have indicated a risk 2-fold increased of nonfatal VTE with use of HCs containing desogestrel or gestodene compared with LNG.Therefore, these studies not provide evidence for a cause-and-effect relationship between HCs- containing desogestrel or gestodene and VTE. Enhancement by thrombophilic diseases ,especially with factor V Leiden mutation of risk of deep-vein-thrombosis associated with oral contraceptives containing a third –generation progestagen has been reported(62,66,82,90, 92). Until now, no sufficient and adequate data about the new formulations as patch, vaginal ring and combined hormonal contraceptives containing progestins with antiandrogenic properties were obtained.

BLOOD HYPERTENSION

Short-term studies have been suggested that combined hormonal contraceptives may induce a mild rise in blood pressure(95,96,97). In fact, it seems that HCs induce hypertension in approximately 5% of users of high-dose pill that contains at least 50 µg estrogen and 1 to 4 mg progestin, however small increases in blood pressure have been reported even among users of modern low-dose formulations(7,97). In fact, it seems that low-dose pill users have a 1. 0 mm Hg rise in diastolic pressure, which is statistically significant but clinically unimportant(99). In addition, blood pressure differences between HC users and non users tend to increase with age.Furthermore, obesity,family history of hypertension and previous hypertensive disorders of pregnancy seem associated with an increase of blood pressure during hormonal contraceptive use(9,100). It is very likely that blood pressure undergoes physiologic variation depending on hormonal fluctuations

(96,101,102). Data on long- term and withdrawal effects of HC use on this outcome are, however , scarce. A recent prospective cohort study carried out on HC-users and past users aged 28-75 years, showed that hormonal contraceptives increase blood pressure, and urinary albumin excretion (UAE) and may be deleterious on urinary function in 6.3% of the users. Although stopping may result in correction of these effects.In fact, women who take HCs have an increased risk of developing new hypertension, which returns to baseline within 1 to 3 months of HC cessation(103).Therefore, some cases of irreversible hypertension ,kidney failure and malignant nephrosclerosis have been reported(104,105) Women with pre-existing hypertension who take HCs have an increased risk of stroke and myocardial infarction when compared with hypertensive women who do not(8,61,106)Women who smoke, have an increased risk of hypertension(2 to 3 times)when take HCs .Smoking increases the risk of vascular damage by increasing sympathetic tone, platelet stickness and reactivity,free radical production, damage of endothelium, and by surges in arterial pressure. Surprisingly, this increased risk declines on quitting cigarettes within 2 to 3 months (107. Blood pressure elevations are usually attributed to the estrogen,but there is evidence of a progestin role as well(102,103) The mechanism by which some HCs users develop hypertension is poorly understood,but it may be related to changes in the renin-angiotensin-aldosterone system (108109)The raise of hypertension often associated with raise of weight is the consequence of increased fluid retention in women taking hormonal contraceptives, especially if over 35 years. Androgenic progestins accentuate sodium retention,which may play an important role(110). A short term study showed in women aged 35-39,treated with gestodene 75 mcg/ EE 20 mcg versus gestodene 60 mcg/ EE 15 mcg a non statistically significant mean increase of 4mmHg for systolic pressure and 2 mm Hg for diastolic pressure in the first group and corresponding increases of 3 and 2 mmHg in the second group(110). Among young women, HDL cholesterol levels decline and LDL levels increase among users relative nonusers of HCs. On the other hand,old women treated with estrogens have more favorable lipid profiles than do women of the same age not receiving estrogen(26). Considering the role of renin-angiotensin-aldosterone system in the development of hypertension,it is possible to explain the absence of effects on hypertension exerted by progestins containing HCs with antiandrogenic properties and, particularly of the drospirenone, an aldosterone- derivative(110,111,112). Although the first problem is the HC prescription and following use with prevalence of uncontrolled hypertension (113).In fact, women with hypertension should be cautioned about the effects of estrogen-containing oral contraceptives which may cause a further elevation in systemic blood pressure. Women with hypertension are at increased risk for cardiovascular events. HC users who did not have their blood pressure measured before initiating HC use were at higher risk for ischemic stroke and myocardial infarction, but not for haemorrhagic stroke or VTE, than HC users who did have their blood pressure measured(2,7,8).

In the meantime,in order to evaluate the risk factors for VTE and cardiovascular disease, prior to the prescription of combined hormonal contraceptives a full clinical, personal and family history,together with the measure of blood pressure and body mass index(BMI) may be advisable.

REFERENCES

[1] Jordan, W. M.(1961). Pulmonary embolism. *Lancet*, II, 1146-7
[2] Tanis, B. C., Rosendaal, F.R. (2003).Venous and arterial thrombosis during oral contraceptive use: risks and risk factors .*Semin .Vasc.Med*, 3(1),69-84.)
[3] Throrogood, M. (1997). Oral contraceptives and myocardial infarction:new evidence leaves unanswered questions. *Thromb.Haemost*, 78(1), 334-8.
[4] Khader, Y.S., Rice, J.J.L., Abueita, O. (2003). Oral contraceptives use and risk of myocardial infarction: a meta-analysis. *Contraception*, 68, 11-7
[5] Kelleher, C.C. (1991). Cardiovascular risks of oral contraceptives: dose-response relationship.Contracept. Fertil. *Sex*, 19(4), 285-8
[6] Lidegaard, O. (1999). Smoking and use of oral contraceptives:impact on thrombotic diseases.*Am.J.Obstet. Gynecol*, 180(6), S 357-63
[7] Hannaford, P. (2000). Cardiovascular events associated with different combined oral contraceptives: a review of current data. *Drug Saf*, May, 22(5), 361-71.
[8] Curtis, K.M., Mohllajee, A.P., Martins, S.L., Peterson, H.B. (2006). Combined oral contraceptives use among women with hypertension: a systematic review. *Contraception*, 73(2), 179-88.
[9] Nessa, A., Latif, S.A., Siddiqui, N.I. (2006). Risk of cardiovascular diseases with oral contraceptives. *Mymensingh. Med. J*, 15(2), 220-4
[10] Tanis, B.C., Bloemenkamp, D.G.,Van den Bosch, M.A., Kemmeren, J.M., Algra, A.,Van de Graaf, Y., Rosendaal, F.R. (2003). Prothrombotic coagulation defects and cardiovascular risk factors in young women with acute myocardial infarction. *Br.J.Haematol*, 122(3), 471-8.
[11] Petitti, D.B., Sidney, S., Quesenberry, C.P. (1998). Oral contraceptive use and myocardial infarction. *Contraception*, 57(3), 143-55.
[12] Mann, J.I., Inman, W.H. (1975).Oral contraceptives and death from myocardial infarction. *Br.Med.J*, 2(5965), 245-8.
[13] Lewis, H.A., Heinemann, L.A., Spitzer, W.O., MacRae, K.D., Bruppacher, R. (1997). The use of oral contraceptives and the occurrence of acute myocardial infarction in young women. Results from the Transnational Study on Oral Contraceptives and the Health of Young Women. *Contraception*, 56(3), 129-40

[14] Sidney, S., Petitti, D.B.,Quesenberry C.P. Jr., Klatsky, A.L., Ziel, H.K.,Wolf, S. (1996). Myocardial infarction in users of low-dose oral contraceptives.*Obstet.Gynecol*, 88(6), 939-44.)
[15] Rosendaal, F.R., Helmerhorst, F.M., Vandenbroucke, J.P. (2002). Female hormones and thrombosis. *Arterioscler. Thromb.Vasc.Biol*, 22(2), 201-10.
[16] Kuhl, H. (1997).Effects of progestogens on haemostasis.Maturitas1996, 24. *Myocardial Infarction and Oral Contraceptives Study*.
[17] Beigbeder, J.Y., Klouche, K., Gallay, P., Levy, G., Grolleau, R. (1990). Myocardial infarction and anti-ethinylestradiol antibody.A propos of a case in an 18-year –old woman.Arch.Mal.*Coeur Vaiss*, 83(7), 1015-8.
[18] Orti, G., Mira, Y.,Vaya, A. (2007). Acute myocardial infarction associated with Yasmin oral contraceptive .*Clin. Appl. Thromb. Hemost*, 13(3), 336-710.
[19] Benacerraf, A.,Veron, P., Morin, B.,Castillo-Fenoy, A.,Chapuis, A., Ziskind, B. (1977). Myocardial infarction following administration of oral contraceptive agents: 3 cases.Nouv.*Press Med*, 6(1), 22-6.
[20] Lidegaard, O. (1987). Cerebrovascular deaths before and after the appearance of oral contraceptives. *Acta Neurol. Scand,* 75(6), 427-33 .
[21] Ciccone, A., Melis, M. (2003). Ischemic stroke risk in oral contraceptive users. *Stroke,* 34(12), 12 and 231.
[22] Ciccone, A., Gatti, A., Melis, M., Cossu, G., Boncoraglio, G.,Carriero, M.R., Iurlaro, S., Agostoni, E. (2005). Cigarette smoking and risk of cerebral sinus thrombosis in oral contraceptive users:a case-control study. *Neurol.Sci*, 26(5), 319-23.
[23] Kemmeren 2002,Etminan, M. ,Takkouche, B., Isorna, F.C., Samii, A. (2005). Risk of ischaemic stroke in people with migraine: systematic review and meta-analysis of observational studies.*BMJ*, 330, 63-6 .
[24] Ischaemic stroke and combined oral contraceptives: results of an international, multicentre, case-control study. (1996). WHO Collaborative Study of Cardiovascular Disease and Steroid Hormone Contraception. *Lancet,* 348(9026), 498-505.
[25] Haemorrhagic stroke, overall stroke risk, and combined oral contraceptives:results of an international,multicentre,case-control study. (1996).WHO Collaborative Study of Cardiovascular Disease and Steroid Hormone Contraception.*Lancet,* 348(9026), 505-10.
[26] Lidegaard, O. (1995). Decline in cerebral thromboembolism among young women after introduction of low-dose oral contraceptives :an incidence study for the period 1980-1993. *Contraception*, 52(2), 85-92).

[27] Lagosky, S., Witten, C.M. (1993). A case of cerebral infarction in association with free protein S deficiency and oral contraceptive use. *Arch.Phys.Med.Rehabil*, 74(1), 98-100.
[28] Nagumo K,Fukushima T,Takahashi H,Sakakibara Y,Kojima S,Akikusa B. (2007).Thyroid crisis and protein C deficiency in a case of superior sagittal sinus thrombosis. *Brain Nerve*, 59(3), 271-6.
[29] Pruissen, D.M., Slooter, A.J., Rosendaal, F.R., Van der Graaf, Y., Algra, A. (2008). Coagulation factor XIII gene variation,oral contraceptives,and risk of ischemic stroke. *Blood*, 111(3), 1282-6.
[30] Pezzini, A., Grassi, M., Iacovello, L., Del Zotto, E., Archetti, S., Glossi, A., Padovani, A. (2007). Inherited thrombophilia and stratification of ischaemic risk among users of oral contraceptives. *J. Neurol. Neurosurg. Psychiatry*, 78(3), 271-6.
[31] Slooter, A.J., Rosendaal, F.R.,Tanis, B.C., Kemmeren, J.M.,Van der Graaf, Y., Algra, A. (2005). Prothrombotic conditions,oral contraceptives, and the risk of ischemic stroke. *J.Thromb.Haemost*, 3(6), 1213-1217
[32] Green, D. (2003). Thrombophilia and stroke. *Top Stroke Rehabil*, 10(3), 21-33.
[33] Li, Y., Zhou, L.,Coulter, D., Gao, E., Sun, Z., Liu, Y., Wang, X. (2006). Prospective cohort study of the association between use of low-dose oral contraceptives and stroke in Chinese women. Pharmacoepidemiol. *Drug Saf*, 15(10),726-34.
[34] Schwartz, S. M., Siscovick, D.S., Longstreth, W.T., Psaty, B. M., Beverly, R. K., Raghunathan, T.E., Lin, D. (1997). Use of Low –Dose Oral Contraceptives and Stroke in a Young Women. *Annals Int. Med*, Vol.127 Issue 8(part 1), 596-603).
[35] Pareja, A., Láinez, J.M. (1995). Ictus, pregnancy and contraception. *Rev Neurol*, 23 Suppl 1, S87-90
[36] Beral, V., Hermon, C., Kay, C., Hannaford, P., Darby, S., Reeves, G. (1999). Mortality associated with oral contraceptive use:25 year follow- up of cohort of 46.000 women from Royal College of General Practitioners: oral contraception study.*B.M.J*, 318(7176), 96-100.
[37] Thorogood, M., Mann, J., Murphy, M.,Vessey, M. (1992). Fatal stroke and use of oral contraceptives: findings from a case-control study.*Am.J.Epidemiol*, 136(1), 35-45.
[38] Gillum, L.A., Johnston, S.C. (2004). Oral contraceptives and stroke risk: the debate continues. *Lancet Neurol*, 3(8), 453-4.
[39] Frigerio, R., Santoro, P., Ferrarese, C., Agostinoni, E. (2004). Migrainous cerebral infarction:case reports. *Neurol.Sci*, 25(3), S 300-1.

[40] Schwaag, S., Nabavi, D.G., Frese, A., Husstedt, I.W., Evers, S. (2003). The association between migraine and juvenile stroke:a case-control study.*Headache*, 43(2), 90-5

[41] MacClellan, L.R.,Giles, W., Cole, J., Wozniak, M., Stern, B., Mitchell, B.D., Kittner, S.J. (2005). Probable migraine with visual aura and risk of ischemic stroke:the stroke prevention in young women study. *Stroke,* 38(9), 2438-45, 330(7482), 63.

[42] Baillargeon, J.P., Mc Clish, D.K., Essah, P.A., Nestler, J.E. (2005). Association between the current use of low-dose oral contraceptives and cardiovascular arterial disease: a meta-analysis. *J.Clin. Endocrinol.Metab*, 90(7), 3853-70.

[43] Moretti,G., Manzoni, G.C., Carpeggiani, P., Parma, M. (1998). Transitory ischemic attacks,migraine and progestogen drugs.Etiopathogenetic correlations.*Minerva Med*, 71(30), 2125-9.

[44] Cole, J.A., Norman, H., Doherty, M., Walker, A.M. (2007).Venous thromboembolism,myocardial infarction,and stroke among transdermal contraceptive system users. *Obstet.Gynecol*, 109(2), 339-46.

[45] Godsland, I.F.,Winkler, U., Lidegaard, O., Crook, D. (2000).Occlusive vascular diseases in oral contraceptive users. Epidemiology, pathology and mechanisms. *Drugs*, 60(4), 721-869

[46] Heinemann, L.A. (2000). Emerging evidence on oral contraceptives and arterial disease. *Contraception*, 62(2), 29S-36S.

[47] Novotnà, M., Unzeitig, V., Novotny, T. (2002). Arterial diseases in women using combined hormonal contraceptives. *Ceska Gynekol*, 67(3), 157-63.

[48] Holzer, G., Koschat, M.A., Kickinger, W., Clementi, W., Holzer, L.A., Metka, M.M. (2007). Reproductive factors and lower extremity arterial occlusive disease in women.*Eur.J.Epidemiol*, 22(8), 505-11.

[49] Barton, M., Dubey, R.K., Traupe, T. (2002). Oral contraceptives and the risk of thrombosis and atherosclerosis. *Expert Opiun. Investing.Drugs*, 11(3), 329-32

[50] Van Den Bosch, M.A., Kemmeren, J.M.,Tanis, B.C., Mali, W.P., Helmerhorst, F.M., Rosendal, F.R., Algra, A.,Van Der Graaf,Y. (2003). The RATIO study: oral contraceptives and the risk of peripheral arterial disease in young women. *J.Thromb. Haemost*, 1(3), 439-44.

[51] De Maat, M.P., Bladbjerg, E.M., Kluft, C.,Winkler, U.M., Rekers, H., Skouby, S.O., Jespersen, J. (2006). Estrogen receptor 1 haplotype does not regulate oral contraceptive-induced changes in haemostasis and inflammation risk factors for venous and arterial thrombosis. *Hum.Reprod*, 21(6), 1473-6.

[52] Khoda, J., Lantsberg, L., Sebbag, G. (1992). Isolated popliteal artery occlusion in the young. *J.Cardiovasc. Surg*, 33(5), 625-8.
[53] Panzere, C., Brieke, A., Brauer, B., Eggemann, F., Becker, H.M., Dieterie, P. (1998). A young patient with multiple arterial occlusions. *Med.Klin*.(Munich), 93(5), 311-8..
[54] Rozenbaum, H. (1985). Progestins and arterial disease. *Contracept. Fertil.Sex* (Paris), 13(1), 344-55.
[55] Rozenbaum H. (1983). Sex steroids and vascular risk. *Coeur*, 14(1), 91-102.
[56] Schved, J. F., Biron, C. (2002). Progestogens, coagulation and vascular tone. *Gynecol. Obstet. Fertil*, 30(5), 41
[57] Schindler, A.E. (2003). Differential effects of progestins on hemostasis. *Maturitas,* 46, 531-7
[58] Pau, H., Carney, A.S., Walker, R., Murty, G.E. (2000). Is oestrogen therapy justified in the treatment of hereditary haemorrhagic telangiectasia?:a biochemical evaluation. *Clin Otolaryngol Allied Sci*, 25(6), 547- 50
[59] Herkert, O., Kuhl, H., Sandow, J., Busse, R., Schini – Kerth, V.B. (2001).Sex-steroids used in hormonal treatment increase vascular procoagulant activity by inducing thrombin receptor (PAR-1) expression:role of the glucocorticoid receptor. *Circulation*, 104(23), 2826-31.
[60] Robert Ebadi, H., Boehlen, F., de Moerloose, P. (2007).Inherited thrombophilia and arterial diseases. *Rev Med Suisse*, Feb 7, 3(97), 331-2, 334-5. Review.
[61] Ageno, W., Squizzato, A., Garcia, D., Imberti, D. (2006). Epidemiology and risk factors of venous thromboembolism.*Semin Thromb Hemost*, Oct, 32(7), 651-8. Review.
[62] Brouwer, J.L., Veeger, N.J., Kluin-Nelemans, H.C., van der Meer, J. (2006).The pathogenesis of venous thromboembolism: evidence for multiple interrelated causes. *Ann Intern Med*, Dec 5, 145(11), 807-15.
[63] MacGillavry, M.R., Prints, M.I.L. (2003).Oral contraceptives and inherited trombophilia :a gene-environment interaction with a risk of venous thrombosis?*Semin.Thromb. Hemost*, 29, 219-26.
[64] Blickstein, D., Blickstein, I. (2007). Oral contraception and thrombophilia. *Curr.Opin.Obstet.Gynecol*, 19(4), 370-6.
[65] Van Vlijmen, E.F., Brouwer, J.L., Veeger, N.J., Eskes, T.K., de Graeff, P.A., van der Meer, J. (2007).Oral contraceptives and the absolute risk of venous thromboembolism in women with single or multiple thrombophilic defects: results from a retrospective family cohort study. *Arch Intern Med*, Feb 12, 167(3), 282-9.

[66] Tormene, D., Fortuna, S., Tognin, G., Gavasso, S., Pagnan, A., Prandoni, P., Simioni, P. (2005). The incidence of venous thromboembolism in carriers of antithrombin, protein C or protein S deficiency associated with the HR2 haplotype of factor V: a family cohort study. *J Thromb Haemost*, Jul, 3(7), 1414-20.

[67] Santamaría, A., Mateo, J., Oliver, A., Menéndez, B., Souto, J.C., Borrell, M., Soria, J.M., Tirado, I., Fontcuberta, J. (2001). Risk of thrombosis associated with oral contraceptives of women from 97 families with inherited thrombophilia: high risk of thrombosis in carriers of the G20210A mutation of the prothrombin gene. *Haematologica*, Sep, 86(9), 965-71.

[68] Simonis, G., Schmeisser, A., Strasser, R.H. (2007). Thrombembolism in a young woman witpreviously unrecognized hereditary hemophilia: obtaining a family history is still strongly recommended before starting oral contraceptives.*Dtsch Med Wochenschr*, 132(44), 2327-9.

[69] Sanson, B.J., Simioni, P., Tormene, D., Moia, M., Friederich, P.W., Huisman, M.V., Prandoni, P., Bura, A., Rejto, L., Wells, P., Mannucci, P.M., Girolami, A., Büller, H.R., Prins, M.H. (1999). The incidence of venous thromboembolism in asymptomatic carriers of a deficiency of antithrombin, protein C, or protein S: a prospective cohort study. *Blood*, Dec 1, 94(11), 3702-6. 52)

[70] De Stefano, V., Simioni, P., Rossi, E., Tormene, D., Za, T., Pagnan, A., Leone, G. (2006). The risk of recurrent venous thromboembolism in patients with inherited deficiency of natural anticoagulants antithrombin, protein C and protein S. *Haematologica*, May, 91(5), 695-853)

[71] Akkawat, B., Rojnuckarin, P. (2005). Protein S deficiency is common in a healthy Thai population. *J Med Assoc Thai*, Sep, 88 Suppl 4, S249-54. 53)

[72] Comp, P.C., Rsmon, C.T. (1984).Recurrent venous thromboembolism in patients with a partial deficiency of protein S. *N. Engl.J.Med*, 311, 1525-1528.

[73] Key, J.D., Hammill, W.W., Everett, L. (1992). Pulmonary embolus in an adolescent on oral contraceptives. *J.Adolesc.Health*, 13(8), 713-5.

[74] Takami, H., Fukushima, K., Takizawa, M., Kodama, T., Uozumi, H., Kobayakawa, N., Takeuchi, H., Aoyagi, T. (2007). Protein C deficiency manifested as pulmonary aretery thromboembolism induced by oral contraceptive.*Nippon Naika Gakkai Zasshi*, Feb 10, 96(2), 341-3.

[75] Kobayashi, R., Yamashita, A., Gohra, H., Furukawa, S., Oda, T., Hamano, K. (2007). Pulmonary and deep vein thrombosis in a young patient with protein S deficiency: report of a case. *Surg Today*, 37(8), 660-3.

[76] Gerstman, B.B., Piper, J.M., Tomita, D.K., Ferguson, W.J., Stadel, B.V., Lundin, E.E. (1991). Oral contraceptive estrogen dose and the risk of deep venous thromboembolic disease *Am.J. Epidemiol*, 133, 32-37.

[77] Bosma, J., Rijbroek, A., Rauwerda, J.A. (2007). A rare case of thromboembolism in a 21-year old female with elevated factor VIII. *Eur. J. Vasc. Endovasc. Surg*, 34(5), 592-4.

[78] Tirado, I., Mateo, J., Soria, J.M., Oliver, A., Martínez-Sánchez, E., Vallvé, C., Borrell, M., Urrutia, T., Fontcuberta, J. (2005). The ABO blood group genotype and factor VIII levels as independent risk factors for venous thromboembolism.*Thromb Haemost*, Mar, 93(3), 468-74.

[79] Conard, J., Plu-Bureau, G., Bahi, N., Horellou, M.H., Pelissier, C., Thalabard, J.C. (2004). Progestogen-only contraception in women at high risk of venous thromboembolism.*Contraception*, Dec,70(6), 437-41.

[80] Belisch, J., Eliakim, V. (1993). Third generation progestagens.Contracept. Fertil. *Sex* (Paris), 21(4), 287-93).

[81] World Health Organisation Collaborative Study of Cardiovascular Disease and Steroid Hormone Contraception. Effect of different progestagens in low estrogen oral contraceptives on venous thromboembolic disease. (1995). *Lancet*, 346, 1582-1588)

[82] Martinez, F., Avecilla, A. (2007). Combined hormonal contraception and venous thromboembolism. *Eur. J .Contracept.Reprod.Health Care,* 12(2), 97-106.

[83] Kemmeren, J.M., Algra, A., Meijers, J.C., Bouma, B.N.,Grobbee, D.E. (2002). Effect of second-and third-generation oral contraceptives on fibrinolysis in the absence or presence of the factor V Leiden mutation. *Blood Coagul Fibrnolysis*, 13(5), 37363)

[84] Aparicio, C., Dahlback, B. (1996). Molecular mechanisms of activated protein C resistance :properties of factor V isolated from an individual with homozygosity for the Arg506 to Gln mutation in the factor V gene. *Biochem. J,* 313, 467-472.

[85] Rosing, J., Tans, G., Nicolaes, G.A. et al. (1997). Oral contraceptives and venous thrombosis: different sensitivities to activated protein C in women using second-and third-generation oral contraceptives. *Br.J Haematol*, 97, 233-238.

[86] Alhenc-Gelas, M., Plu-Bureau, G., Guillonneau, S., Kirzin, J.M., Aiach, M., Ochat, N., Scarabin, P.Y. (2004). Impact of progestagens on activated protein C (APC) resistance among users of oral contraceptives. *J Thromb Haemost*, Sep, 2(9), 1594-600.

[87] Farmer, R.D., Lawrenson, R.A., Thompson, C.R., Kennedy, J.G., Hambleton, I.R. (1997). Population-based study of risk of venous thromboembolism associated with various oral contraceptives. *Lancet*, 349(9045), 83-8.
[88] Jick, H., Jick, S.S.,Gurewich, V., Myers, M.W., Vasilakis, C. (1995). Risk of idiopathic cardiovascular death and nonfatal thrombo embolism in women using oral contraceptives with differing progestagen components. *Lancet*, 346(8990), 1589-93.
[89] Wiegratz, I., Lee, J.H., Kutschera, E.,Winkler, U.H., Kuhl, H. (2004). Effect of four oral contraceptives on hemostatic parameters.*Contraception*, 70(2), 97-106.
[90] Jick, S.S., Kaye, J.A., Russmann, S., Jick, H. (2006). Risk of nonfatal thromboembolism with oral contraceptives containing norgestimate or desogestrel compared with oral contraceptives containing levonorgestrel. *Contraception*, 73(6), 566-70.
[91] Bloemenkamp, K.W., Rosendaal, F.R., Helmerhorst, F.M., Buller, H.R.,Vandenbroucke, J.P. (1995). Enhancement by factor V Leiden mutation of risk of deep-vein-thrombosis associated with oral contraceptives containing a third –generation progestagen. *Lancet*, 346 (8990:1593-6).
[92] Norris, L.A., Bonnar, J. (1996). The effect of oestrogen dose and progestogen type on haemostatic changes in women taking low dose oral contraceptives. *Br.J.Obstet.Gynecol*, 103(3), 261-7.
[93] Gerstman, B.B., Piper, J.M., Tomita, D.K., Ferguson, W.J., Stadel, B.V., Lundin, E.E. (1991). Oral contraceptive estrogen dose and the risk of deep venous thromboembolic disease. *Am.J. Epidemiol*, 133, 32-37.
[94] Aldrighi, J.M., De Campos, L.S., Eluf Gebara, O.C., Petta, C.A., Bahamondes, L. (2006). Effect of acombined oral contraceptive containing 20 microg ethinylestradiol and 75 microg gestodene on hemostatic parameters. *Gynecol. Endocrinol*, 22(1), 1-4.
[95] Samlaska, C.P., James, W.D. (1990). Superficial thrombophlebitis II .Secondary hypercoagulable states. *J.Am.Acad.Dermatol*, 23(1), 1-18
[96] Kluft, C., Meijer, P., Laguardia, K.D., Fisher, A.C. (2008). Comparison of a transdermal patch vs .oral contraceptives on hemostasis variables. *Contraception*, 77(2), 77-83.
[97] Chasan –Taber, L., Willet, W.C., Manson, J. E., Spiegelman, D., Hunter, D. J., Curhan, G., Colditz, G.A., Stampfer, M. J. (1996). Prospective study of oral contraceptives and hypertension among women in the United States.*Circulation*, 94(3), 483-9.

[98] Naruse, M.,Tanabe, A. (2006). Estrogen –induced hypertension .*Nippon Rinsho*, 3, 504-8.
[99] Carr, B.R., Ory, H. (1997). Estrogen and progestin components of oral contraceptives :relationship to vascular disease. *Contraception,* 55(5), 267-72.
[100] Shen, Q., Lin, D., Jiang, X., Li, H., Zhang, Z. (1994). Blood pressure changes and hormonal contraceptives. *Contraception,* 50(2), 131-141.
[101] Narkiewicz, K., Graniero, G.R., D'Este, D., Mattarei, M., Zonzin, P., Palatini, P. (1995). Ambulatory blood pressure in mild hypertensive women taking oral contraceptives. A case-control study. *Am. J. Hypertens,* 8(3), 249-53.
[102] Dong, W., Colhoun, H.M., Poulter, N.R. (1997). Blood pressure in women using oral contraceptives: results from the Health Survey for England 1994. *J. Hypertens*, 15(10), 1063-8
[103] Morley Kotchen, J., Kotchen, T.A. (2003). Impact of female hormones on blood pressure: review of potential mechanisms and clinical studies.*Curr.Hypertens.Rep*, 5(6), 505-12.
[104] Atthobari, J., Gansevoort, R.T., Visser, S.T., De Jong, P.E., De Jong –van den Berg, L.T. (2007). Prevend StudyGroup. The impact of hormonal contraceptives on blood pressure, urinary albumin excretion and glomerular filtration rate. *Br. J. Clin. Pharmacol*, 63(2), 224-31.
[105] Lin, K.G., Isies, C.G., Hodsman, G.P., Lever, A.F., Robertson, J.W. (1987). Malignant hypertension in women of childbearing age and its relation to the contraceptive pill. *Br. Med. J.* (Clin. Res. Ed.), 294 (6579), 1057-9.
[106] Riera, M., Navas –Parejo, A., Gomez, M., Cerezo, S. (2004). Malignant hypertension and irreversible kidney failure associated with oral contraception pill intake. *Nefrologia*, 24(3), 298-9.
[107] Pollara, T., Kelsberg, G., Safranek, S., Schrager, S. (2006). Clinical inquiries. What is the risk of adverse outcomes in a woman who develops mild hypertension from Oc s? *J.Fam. Pract*, 55(11), 986-8.
[108] Sleight, P. (1993). Smoking and hypertension. *Clin. Exp. Hypertens*, 15(6), 1181-92.
[109] Ribstein, J., Halimi, J.M.,du Cailar, G., Mimran, A. (1999). Renal characteristics and effect of angiotensin suppression in oral contraceptive users.*Hypertension*, Jan, 33(1), 90-5.
[110] Singh, H., Schwartzman, M.L. (2008). Renal vascular cytochrome P450-derived eicosanoids in androgen-induced hypertension. *Pharmacol.Rep*, 60(1), 29-37.

[111] Pechère-Bertachi, A., Maillard, M., Staider, H., Biscof, P., Fathi, M., Brunner, H.R., Burnier, M. (2003). Renal hemodynamic responses to salt in women using oral contraceptives. *Kidney Int,* 64(4), 1374-80.
[112] De Leo, V., La Marca, A., Morgante, G., Lucani, B., Nami, R.,Ciotta, L., Cianci, A., Petraglia, F. (2001). Evaluation of plasma levels of renina-aldosterone and blood pressure in women over 35 years treated with new oral contraceptives. *Contraception,* 64(3), 145-8.
[113] Oelkers, W., Foidart, J.M., Dombrovicz, N.,Welter, A., Heithecker, R. (1995). Effects of a new oral contraceptive containing an antimineralocorticoid progestogen,drospirenone,on the rennin-aldosterone system,body weight,blood pressure,glucose tolerance,and lipid metabolism. *J. Clin. Endocrinol.Metab,* 80(6), 1816-21.
[114] Lubianca, J.N., Faccin, C.S., Fucchs, F.D. (2003). Oral contraceptives:a risk factor for uncontrolled blood pressare among hypertensive women.*Contraception,* 67(1), 19-24.

PART II, OTHER EFFECTS

Rosa Sabatini
Dept.Obstetrics and Gynecology,
General Hospital Policlinico-University of Bari, Italy

ANGIOEDEMA

Angioedema is a potentially life threatening condition and may be inherited or acquired.According to sporadic reports, hormonal contraceptives can induce or exacerbate symptoms of hereditary angioedema type I or type III or idiopathic angioedema. However, many women with these diseases may use oral contraceptives without having any effect on their angioedema(1). The main symptoms include sudden swilling and reddening of the skin which can improve after hormonal contraceptive (HC) cessation(2).Although in rare cases, patients presenting severe abdominal pain and laryngeal oedema can have airway obstruction and even death(3) It is advisable that clinicians should not administer estrogen-containing contraceptives to women known to have hereditary angioedema, in whom C1-esterase inhibitor (C1 INH)deficiency was demonstrated. In fact,evidence showed a remarkable improvement with increase of C1-INH, after HC discontinuation.Several studies reported that HCs may play an iatrogenic role in the aetiology of chronic angioneurotic oedema or urticaria.(4). Hormonal measurement demonstrated that the number of attacks is significantly higher in female with high progesterone levels;while,a significantly lower attack frequency ,during 1-year follow-up, in patients with a higher (40 nmol/ l) SHBG level(5).Recurrent angioedema is biochemically characterized by reduced C1 inhibitor level and/or function ,and genetically by a heterogeneous group of mutations in the C1 inhibitor gene that have an autosomal dominant mode of trasmission(6). Recently, a new type of hereditary angioedema(type 3) has been reported .This occurs only in women and is characterized by normal C1-INH levels and severe attacks of angioedema,which are clinically indistinguishables from the classic form(7,8,9). Acquired forms of angioedema are estrogen (both endogenous and exogenous)dependent ,although it seems that progesterone-only-contraceptives may also induce attacks of this disease(2,8).

REFERENCES

[1] Bork, K., Fischer, B., Dewald, G. (2003). Recurrent episodes of skin angioedema and severe attacks of abdominal pain induced by oral contraceptives or hormone replacement therapy. *Am. J.Med*, 114(4), 294-8
[2] Yip, J., Cunliffe, W.J. (1992). Hormonally exacerbated hereditary angioedema. Australas.J.Dermatol, 33(1), 35-8
[3] Kumar, M.A., Gupta, C. (2005). Acquired angioedema secondary to hormone replacement therapy. *Indian J.Med.Sci*, 59(10), 451-4
[4] André, C., André, F.,Veysseyre-Balter, C., Rousset, H. (2003). Acquired angioneurotic edema induced by hormonal contraception.*Presse Med*, 32(18), 831-5
[5] Visy, B., Fust, G.,Varga, L., Szendei, G.,Takàcs, E., Karadi, I., Fekete, B., Harmat, G., Farkas, H. (2004). Sex hormones in hereditary angioneurotic oedema. *Clin.Endocrinol*, 60(4), 508-15.
[6] Binkley, K.E., Davis, A.E. (2003). Estrogen-dependent inherited angioedema. *Transfus.Apher.Sci*, 29(3), 215-9.
[7] Van der Klooster, J.M., Schelfhout, L.J.,Grootendorst, A.F., Zweers, P.G. (2002). Recurrent attacks of angioedema ascribed to the use of estrogen preparations and a pregnancy(hereditary angioedema type 3).*Ned.Tijdschr.Geneeskd*, 146(34), 1599-602.
[8] André, F.,Veysseyre-Balter, C., Rousset, H., Descos, L., André, C. Exogenous oestrogen as an alternative to food allergy in the aetiology of angioneurotic oedema.*Toxicology*, 2''3, 185(1-2), 155-60.
[9] Bettoni, L. (2005). Influence of ethinyl estradiol on C1inhibitor:a new etiopathogenesic mechanism of angioedema:case report. *Eur. Ann.Allergy Clin.Immunol*, 37(2), 49.

PELIOSIS HEPATIS

The peliosis hepatis,firstly described in 1950 by Zak F.G., is a rare condition,sometimes fatal, characterized by areas of hepatocellular necrosis secondarily cystic,blood filled cavities of 1-3 mm of diameter in the parenchyma.Initially,only focal hepatocellular necrosis may be present, sometimes hemorrhagic but in the severe and fatal cases, portal hypertension with varices and ascites,liver failure and/ or hemoperitoneum with shock secondary to intraperitoneal rupture were reported(1). Some cases are reported in women taking oral contraceptives.In this circumstance , regression of the initial lesions is possible with termination of the etiologic agent(2,3).This rare disease,generally develops in organs belonging to the mononuclear phagocytic system (liver,spleen, bone marrow,lymph nodes); however,a paucity of studies indicates that other organs such as lungs, parathyroid glands, and kidneys may be affected,too.(4)

REFERENCES

[1] Jacquemin, E., Pariente, D., Fabre, M., Huault, G.,Valayer, J., Bernard, O. (1999). Peliosis hepatis with initial presentation as acute hepatic failure and intraperitoneal hemorrhage in children. *J.Hepatol*, 30(6), 1146-50.
[2] Hung, N.R.,Chantrain, L., Dechambre, S. (2004). eliosis hepatis revealed by biliary colic in a patient with oral contraceptive use. *Acta Chir.Belg*, 104(6), 727-9.
[3] Eugene, M., Chong, M.F., Genin, R., Amat, D. (1985). Peliosis hepatis and oral contraceptives :a case report. *Mediterr. Med*, 13(343), 21-24.
[4] Zafrani, E.S., Pinaudeau, Y., Le Cudonnec, B., Julien, M., Dhumeaux, D. (1980). Focal hemorrhagic necrosis of the liver.A clinicopathological entity possibly related to oral contraceptives. *Gastroenterology*, 79, 1295-9.

SEVERE ADVERSE OCULAR REACTIONS

The incidence of ocular complications from hormonal contraceptives was estimated to be 1 in 230,000 users(1). Therefore, severe adverse vascular accidents of the eye are exceptional in women under 40 years and without risk factors(2). Spasm of the central retinal artery, generally precedes occlusion and requires immediate ophthalmologic examination and discontinuation of COC s.On the contrary, this event lead to loss of sight and functional recuperation in unusual

(3,4,5). In fact, acute retinal arterial vascular occlusive disorders represent the more important cause of blindness or serious impaired vision ; although, their pathogenesis is hitherto a controversial issue(6,7).

Venous occlusion occurs less suddenly and involves a less extensive loss of sight.The prognosis depends on the affected area. Symptomatology of the ophthalmic vein thrombosis may be variable: unilateral proptosis,haemorrhagic retinopathy and,increase in intraocular pressure can be differently associated.There is a complete resolution of the vein thrombosis and eye signs and symptoms with the discontinuation of the hormonal contraceptive(8).Therefore, these worned vascular effects in women taking hormonal contraceptives are very rare(9,10)The risk is affected by smoking, irregular lipid and glucose metabolism,and hypertension.Although ocular complications are unusual,they should be kept in mind and women with a history of vascular problems,visual problems ,or migraines should be excluded before COCs are prescribed.Particularly, migraine should be considered a warning signal (11) Retinal disorders have been more common in women who complained of headache .However, the incidence of these complications seems to lesser with the estrogen -dose reduction and the use of third-generation progestins (12). Other conditions as the isolated retinal bleeding and vascular papillitis,are reversed on termination of COCs use.The more rare macular edema have been reported but the data resulted insufficient to permit a casuality relationship with COCs. Retrobulbar optic neuropathy in young women may be considered as the first manifestation of a sclerosis. Ophthalmic migraines are,also,reported in sporadic cases(13). However, experimental studies on the ocular effects of oral contraceptives in animals showed only increased permeability of the lens and possibly vascular dilatation(14). Possible aetiopathogenetic interrelations between hormonal contraceptives and ocular side-effects are still controversial; however, when the HC –user reports a vision decrease or persistent or recurrent headache it is convenient that hormonal contraception is discontinued(15).

REFERENCES

[1] Leff, S.P. (1976). Side-effects of oral contraceptives:occlusion of branch artery of the retina. *Bull.Sinai Hosp. Detroit*, 24(4), 227-9.
[2] Rekhi, G.S., Dheer, S. (2002). Oral contraceptive-induce central retinal artery occlusion. *J. Assoc. Phisicians India*, 50,1084-5.
[3] Mehta, C. (1999).Central retinal artery occlusion and oral contraceptives. *Indian J. Ophthalmol*, 47(1), 35-6.

[4] Blade, J., Darleguy, P., Chanteau, Y. (1971). Early thrombosis of the retinal artery and oral contraceptives. *Bull. Soc. Ophtalmol*, 71(1), 48-9.
[5] Girolami, A., Vettore, S., Tezza, F., Girolami, B. (2007). Retinal central artery occlusion in a young woman after ten days of a drospirenone-containing oral contraceptive. *Thromb. Haemost*, 98(2), 473-4.
[6] Hayreh, S.S. (2005). Prevalent misconceptions about acute retinal vascular occlusive disorders. *Prog.Retin. Eye Res*, 24 (4), 493-519.
[7] Blade, J., Darleguy, P., Chanteau, Y. (1971). Early thrombosis of the retinal artery and oral contraceptives. *Bull. Soc. Ophtalmol*, 71(1), 48-9.
[8] Jaais, F., Habib, Z.A. (1994).Unilateral superior ophthalmic vein thrombosis in a user of oral contraceptives. *J. Med. Malaysia*, 49(4), 416-8.
[9] Villatte-Cathelineau, B. (1985).The eye and hormones:vascular disorders associated with combined oral contraceptives and pregnancy. *Contracept.Fertil. Sex(Paris)*, 13(1), 147-52.
[10] Villatte-Cathelineau, B. (1985). The eye and hormones:vascular disorders associated with combined oral contraceptives and pregnancy. *Contracept.Fertil. Sex(Paris)*, 13(1), 147-52.
[11] Asensio Sànchez, V.M., Pèrez Flandez, F.J., Bartolomè Aragon, A., Gil Fernandez, E. (2002). Ophthalmologic vascular occlusions and oral contraceptives.*Arch. Soc.Esp. Oftalmol*, 77(3), 163-6
[12] Glacet-Bernard, A., Kuhn. D., Soubrane, G. (1999). Ocular complications of hormonal treatments:oral contraception and menopausal hormonal replacement therapy. *Contracept.Fertil.Sex*, 27(4), 285-90.
[13] Hayreh, S.S. (2005). Prevalent misconceptions about acute retinal vascular occlusive disorders. *Prog.Retin. Eye Res*, 24(4), 493-519.
[14] Malek, N., Lebuisson, D.A. (1992).Adverse ocular reactions to oral contraceptive use. *Contracept. Fertil. Sex(Paris)*, 20(4), 441-4.
[15] Wood, J.R. (1977). Ocular complications of oral contraceptives.*Ophthalmic.Semin*, 2(4), 371-402.

VASCULITIS

Some studies affirmed that hormonal contraceptves,sometimes may provoke vasculitis. Since Kussmaul and Maier described the index case of vasculitis in 1866, the field has seen many changes but many mysteries remain (1). Vasculitis represent such a heterogeneous group of disorders which may involve small arteries, arterioles, capillaries,and venules(2,3).Cutaneous vasculitis may be confined to the skin or may be part of an associated systemic disease (4) .Oral contraceptives (OCs) can affect the skin through their hormonal effects or through iatrogenic effects associated with their toxicity in certain individuals. Toxic effects of OCs are rare but potentially serious; they should be diagnosed early and require permanent termination of OC use. The clinical manifestations are variable and not specific to the medication. The most frequently reported manifestations are allergic vascularities which may lead to serious renal complications, fixed pigmented erythema, urticaria, and lichenoid eruptions (5). Associations between markers of allergy (eosinophils, IgE and atopy) and hormonal dependent events in women (premenstrual asthma, menopause and oral contraceptive use) have been found (6). In women, combined steroid contraceptives caused a decrease in antibody formation and complement levels and exhibited an immunosuppressive effect " in vitro" on lymphocyte activation by nonspecific mitogens. In vivo, the immunosuppressive effect on lymphocytes is evident after approximately 2 years of contraceptive use and, remained for several months after discontinuation of the drug. In women with rheumatoid arthritis who used steroid contraceptives, an improvement in symptoms occured; in unaffected women, the risk for acquiring the disease was decreased by half. There was an improvement in the symptoms of chronic bronchial asthma, but there were also, some cases of allergic manifestations 1 to 2 months after beginning contraceptive use (7). Contradictory results were reported on the effect of steroid contraceptives on allergic diseases in women. Clinical manifestation ranging from vessel hypersensitivity and allergic angitis to other forms of vasculitis indistinguishables from classical systemic forms as Wegener's granulomatosis, polyarteritis nodosa or Churg-Strauss syndrome (8, 9,10).Half of the patients with Wegener's granulomatosis develop skin lesions due to the systemic vasculitis. Differential diagnostic considerations may present several difficulties and a skin biopsy is necessary for establishing the diagnosis. Antineutrophil cytoplasmic antibodies with antigen specificity for proteinase 3 (PR3-ANCA) supports the diagnosis of Wegener granulomatosis(11).Wegener's granulomatosis is an organ- and/or life-threatening autoimmune disease of as yet unknown etiology. The classic clinical triad consists of necrotizing granulomatous inflammation of the upper and/or lower respiratory tract, necrotizing glomerulonephritis, and an autoimmune necrotizing systemic vasculitis affecting predominantly small vessels. The detection of antineutrophil cytoplasmic antibodies directed against proteinase 3 (PR3-ANCA) is highly specific for Wegener's granulomatosis. ANCA positivity is found only in about 50% of the patients with localized Wegener's granulomatosis (which is restricted to the respiratory tract and affects < or = 5% of the patients), whereas PR3-ANCA positivity is seen in 95% of the patients with generalized Wegener's granulomatosis(12).Vasculitis is an independent risk factor for diffuse endothelial dysfunction and may be a consequence of TNF-alpha action on endothelial cells(9,10). Polyarteritis nodosa has been progressive illness resulting in a systemic necrotizing vasculitis which may affect the kidneys, gastrointestinal tract, skin, nerves and,muscles .Churg-Strauss is a hypereosinophilic syndrome inducing systemic vasculitis(10).The subjects affected may be tested for the presence of the FIP1L1-PDGRFA mutation(13). In conclusion , hormonal contraceptives may induce allergic vascularities.It is hypotesized as possible etiology a reaction of cell-mediated immunity.Affected subjects may present cutaneous involvement alone or life-threatening systemic involvement,which may result in severe and sometimes fatal illness. Although, oral contraceptives when implicated induce generally mild vasculitis, a rare case of vasculitis with cutaneous necrosis HC- containing levonorgestrel 0.15 µg and ethinylestradiol 0.03 mg related was reported (14)

REFERENCES

[1] Stone, J.H. (2007).Vasculitis:a collection of pearls and myths.*Rheum.Dis.Clin.North Am*,33(4), 691-739.
[2] Youinou, P. (2008). Vasculitis :Current Status and Future Directions. *Clin. Rev. Allergy Immunol.*
[3] Mullick, F.G., McAllister, H.A., Wagner, B.M., Fenoglio, J.J.Jr. (1979). Drug related vasculitis.Clinicopathologic correlations in 30 patients. *Hum.Pathol*, 10(3), 313-25.
[4] Mat,C.,Yurdakul, S.,Tuzuner, N.,Tuzun, Y. (1997). Small vessel vasculitis and vasculitis confined to skin.*Baillieres Clin. Rheumatol*, 11(2), 237-57.
[5] Thomas, P., Dalle, E., Revillon, B., Delecour, M., Devarenne, M.F., Pagniez, I. (1985).Cutaneous effects in hormonal contraception. *NPN Med*, 5(81),19-24
[6] Siroux, V., Oryszczyn, M.P.,Varraso, R., Le Moual, N., Bousquett, J., Charpin, D.,Gormand, F., Kennedy, S., Maccario, J., Pison, C., Rage, E., Scheinmann, P.,Vervioet, D., Pin, I., Kauffman, F. (2007).Environmental factors for asthma severity and allergy.results from the EGEA study. *Rev.Mal.Respir*, 24(5), 599-608
[7] Presl, J. (1982).Steroidal contraceptives and the immune system. *Cesk Gynekol*, 47(2), 599-608.
[8] Lamprecht, P., Gross, W.L. (2004). Wegener's granulomatosis. *Herz*, Feb, 29(1), 47-56.Review.

[9] Bonsib, S.M. (2001). Polyarteritis nodosa. *Semin. Diagn. Pathol*, 18(1), 14-23

[10] Melimich, B., Holl-Ulrich, K., Merz, M.,Gross, W.L. (2007).Hypereosinophilic syndrome andChurg-Strauss syndrome: is it clinically relevant to differentiate these syndromes? *Internist*.(Berl.).

[11] Ben Ghotbel, I., Dhrif, A.S., Miled, M., Houman, M.H. Cutaneous manifestations as the initial presentation of Wegener's granulomatosis.*Presse Med*,36(4 Pt 1), 619-22.

[12] Bounny, C., Nievergelt, H., Braathen, L.R., Simon, D. *Wegener's granulomatosis presenting as pyoderma gangrenosum*. Clinic and Polyclinic for Dermatology, Inselspital, University of Bern , Switzerland.

[13] Levy, S.A., Franca, A.T., De La Reza, D.,Valle, S.O.,Correla, A.H. (2006).Asthma and Churg-Strauss syndrome.*J.Bras.Pneumol*, 32(4), 367-70.

[14] Mosovich, B., Biton, A., Avinoach, I. (1991).Vaculitis with cutaneous necrosis induced by oral contraceptive .*Harefuah*, 120(8), 451-3.

In: Adverse Effects of Hormonal Contraceptives ISBN: 978-1-60692-819-6
Editor: R. Sabatini © 2009 Nova Science Publishers, Inc.

PART III, CANCER RISKS

R. Sabatini[1], P. Trerotoli[2], R. Cagiano[3], M. Tartagni[1] and G. Serio[2]

[1] Department of Obstetrics and Gynecology
[2] Department of.Biomedical Sciences and Human Oncology
[3] Department of.Pharmacology
General Hospital Policlinico-University of Bari, Italy

NEOPLASTIC RISK OF HORMONAL CONTRACEPTION

For several years the role of hormonal contraceptives(HCs) in the development of cancer has been explored, in all countries. Their beneficial effects were well documented, but many questions are still raised concerning a possible connexion with malignant tumours(1,2).

BREAST CANCER RISK

The clinical impact of the association between hormonal contraceptives use and breast cancer risk is very important considering the widespread HCs use and, that more than a quarter of a million women are diagnosed as having breast cancer in the United States, annually (3) Women who are currently combined oral contraceptives(COCs)users or have used them in the past 10 years are at a slightly increased risk of having breast cancer during the next 10 years; although the additional cancers diagnosed tend to be localized to the breast and they are less advanced clinically than the cancers diagnosed in those who have never used

HCs(4). Particular interest was devoted to predisposed women as the BRCA1/BRCA2 mutation carriers; although recent international studies reported in those no evidence that the current use of combined oral contraceptives (COCs) might be associated with a risk more strongly than in the general population. However, duration of use, especially before first full-term pregnancy, may be associated with an increasing risk of breast cancer among both BRCA 1 and BRCA2 mutation carriers(5,6,7). Some researchers have suggested that there may be an increase in the risk of breast cancer associated with a prior induced abortion in users or past users of HCs. The risk, if present, may vary according to the duration of the pregnancy in which the abortion occurred, or to a woman's age or parity at that time,or the age at menarche, and to have used oral contraceptives for an extended period of time. The breast cancer relative risk(RR) in those with one or more induced abortion was 1.2 fold to women with no history of abortion and was reported greatest (2.0) among nulliparous women whose abortion or abortions occurred prior to 8 weeks' gestation(8). This risk was slightly higher when the abortion was performed before 20 years of age or after 29 years of age with a relative risk(RR) of 1.5.The data from these studies do not permit a causal interpretation at this time, nor do they identify any particular subgroup of women with induced abortion histories at enhanced risk of breast cancer(8,9, 10).In general, no association has been found between spontaneous abortion and the risk for breast cancer(1,10).An association between breast cancer and long-term HC use among young women , beginning close to menarche suggests that puberty, a time when breast epithelial cells are undergoing considerable proliferative activity, are susceptible to genetic damage. In addition, the frequency in this age group of imbalances of adrenal-ovarian maturation might have importance

(11,12). Although seems that in younger women baseline risk for breast cancer is extremely low (13). Scarce data are available to assign a risk for progestin-only-pill(11).However,the effects of medroxy- progesterone acetate (MPA)as well as norethisterone (NET) were investigated in the presence of a growth factor mixture and/ or estradiol in normal and neoplastic human epithelial breast cells, and it seems that MPA may increase breast cancer risk in women when used in long-term treatment. In this respect NET reacts neutral. The mitosis of pre-existing cancerous cells may be partly inhibited by the addition of both progestogens(14). Thus, these results indicate that it is necessary to differentiate between normal and malignant breast cells concerning the assessment of progestogens as a risk factor for the breast.Data regarding injected or implanted hormonal contraceptives are limited. However, it seems that implants could induce higher risk for breast cancer than injected preparations (OR 8.59);while, associations between injected HC use and breast cancer in women are consistent with modestly increased risk among recent users and for ER (estrogen receptors)negative tumors. Based on a small number of users of subdermal implant contraceptives in this study, a significant increase in breast cancer risk was observed; continued surveillance of implant users may be warranted(15). Early breast cancer and ovarian cancer screening are recommended for women with BRCA1/2 mutations. Inherited breast and ovarian cancers account for 10% of all breast and ovarian cancers(16).Relative to sporadic breast and ovarian cancers, these cancers tend to occur at an earlier age and grow more aggressively. Identification of patients with the mutation is therefore crucial, because preventive measures such as prophylactic bilateral mastectomy, prophylactic bilateral salpingo-oophorectomy and chemoprevention with Tamoxifen can prevent breast and ovarian cancer(17,18).. Likewise, genetic counseling prior to testing is important, considering the major impact of the test results on an individual's life(19,20) No absolute recommendation is made for or against prophylactic surgery; these surgeries are an option for mutation carriers,but evidence of benefit is lacking,and case reports have documented the occurrence of cancer following prophylactic surgery(21). Many women would prefer fewer bleeding episodes while taking oral contraceptives. For this reason and with the intention of reducing menstruation-associated symptoms, an extended-cycle contraceptive is often considered. The results of a study " in vitro" indicate that continuously administered ethinylestradiol may not increase breast cancer risk in comparison to intermittent application(22). However, it remains unknown whether this long-term treatment is associated with a different breast cancer risk from that of the usual treatment.Another study in vitro assessed the effects of progesterone(P),testosterone(T), chlormadinone acetate (CMA), medroxyprogesterone (MPA), norethisterone(NET),levonorgestrel (LNG), dienogest(DNG),gestodene(GSD) and 3-ketodesogestrel (KDG)in normal human breast epithelial MCF10A cells and in estrogen and progesterone receptor positive HCC1500 human primary breast cancer cells.The results showed that MPA and CMA, with growth factors (GFs), induced proliferation of MCF10A cells. While,P, T, NET, LNG, DNG, GSD and KDG had no significant effect. In HCC1500 cells, MPA and CMA with GFs had an inhibitory effect NET, LNG, DNG, GSD, KDG and T enhanced the proliferative effect of GFs. P had no significant effect. No progestogen could further enhance the stimulatory effect of E2 on HCC1500 cells,all but KDG inhibited it. MPA, GSD, T, CMA and NET had an anti-proliferative effect on the mitotic GF and E2 combination. P, LNG, DNG and KDG had no significant effect. So, some progestogens may induce proliferation or inhibit growth of benign or malignant human breast epithelial cells independently of the effects of growth factors and E2(23). So, choice of progestogen for hormone therapy may be important in terms of influencing possible breast cancer risk.However,clinical studies are necessary to prove these results obtained in vitro.

OVARIAN CANCER RISK

The incidence of ovarian cancer is reduced by pregnancy, lactation, tubal ligation and oral contraceptives(24).The role of sex hormones seems important for ovarian carcinogenesis. Epidemiological observations and experimental data from the animal model indicate that estrogens may have an adverse effect, while progesterone/progestins reduce the effect directly on the ovarian epithelium.There is evidence that oral contraceptive use provides substantial protection against ovarian cancer and that the longer HC use offers the greater reduction in ovarian cancer risk ($p<0.001$)(17,25). However, the eventual public-health effects of this reduction will depend on how long the protection lasts after use ceases. Women who have used oral contraceptives for 5 years or longer , have about half the risk of ovarian cancer compared with never users(26,27, 28). Recently,the Collaborative Group on Epidemiological Studies of Ovarian Cancer (Oxford) reported from a reanalysis of data from 45 epidemiological studies including 23,257 women with ovarian cancer and 87,303 controls that this reduction in risk persisted for more than 30 years after oral contraceptive use had ceased.However,it became somewhat attenuated over time; the proportional risk reductions per 5 years of use were 29% for use that had ceased less than 10 years previously, 19% for use that had ceased 10-19 years previously, and 15% for use that had ceased 20-29 years previously. This effect is not dose-dependent considering the similar proportional risk reduction from the 1960s onwards(29). The incidence of mucinous tumours (12% of the total) seemed little affected by oral contraceptives, but otherwise the proportional risk reduction did not vary much between different histological types. These findings suggest that oral contraceptives have already prevented some 200,000 ovarian cancers and 100,000 deaths from the disease, and that over the next few decades the number of cancers prevented will rise to at least 30,000 per year(18, 29).The reduction of risk does not seem related to androgenicity of the hormonal contraceptives(27,30).Low-estrogen dose oral contraceptives confer a benefit, regarding ovarian cancer risk , similar to that conferred by earlier high-estrogen-dose formulations (31,32,33) While, current available data suggest that long-term use of estrogens may slightly increase the risk, especially of endometrioid type of ovarian cancer(3,30) .The protective effect of combined oral contraceptive pill, was confirmed in multiple studies; however, it is unclear whether this protection also covers women with a genetic predisposition to ovarian cancer or perimenopausal women. About 5% of all ovarian-cancer cases are caused by a genetic predisposition, in particular as a component of the autosomal dominant hereditary breast-ovarian-cancer syndrome. Women with this germline mutations in the cancer susceptibility genes, BRCA1 or BRCA2, have up to an 85% lifetime risk of breast cancer and up to a 46% lifetime risk ovarian cancer(20,31,32).Ovarian and endometrial cancer also occur in families with Lynch/hereditary non-polyposis colorectal cancer syndrome (HNPCC).The syndrome is caused by germline mutations in DNA mismatch-repair genes. Women at high risk of gynaecological cancer based upon familial clustering of disease or a demonstrated pathogenic germ-line mutation are candidates for surveillance: annual gynaecological examinations, including vaginal echoscopy and serum carcinoma antigen CA125 testing. Prophylactic surgery in the form of adnexectomy leads to a marked, but not complete, reduction of ovarian-cancer risk in high-risk cases(17,18,34).There is insufficient evidence to advise against, the use of oral contraceptives or hormonal substitution after adnexectomy for healthy women with a genetic predisposition to breast cancer. Recommendations for surveillance and prevention should be given only after genetic-risk counselling, based on a detailed family study and DNA-based diagnosis (17,18,32). There is emerging evidence that familial breast cancer,including BRCA1 and BRCA2 mutations,could be estrogen sensitive(35). Therefore, endogenous and exogenous estrogens, such as hormonal contraceptives,may increase the risk of breast cancer in BRCA1 mutation carriers.So, HCs, especially,in older women should be used with caution in BRCA1 or BRCA2 mutation carriers(36).

ENDOMETRIAL CANCER RISK

Combination oral contraceptive use was associated with a decreased risk in endometrial carcinoma,which decrease with duration of use (RR=0.28 at 5 years of use);however, the estimated protective effect was reduced and became statistically non-significant when allowance was made for weight and parity (36,37).The benefic effect of HC use was only clearly evident in women who had less than 3 live-births and who had BMI less than 22 kg/m^2(38) .Overall,progestin effect is not dose-dependent; in fact, high progestin potency HCs did not confer significantly more protection than low progestin potency HCs (OR=0.52). However, among women with a body mass index of 22 kg/m^2 or higher, those who used high progestin potency oral contraceptives had a lower risk of endometrial cancer than those who used low progestin potency oral contraceptives(OR=0.31)while those with a BMI below 22.0 kg/m² did not(38,39).A reduced risk of endometrial carcinoma with HCs use was present only among users of five or more years' duration(40). Oral contraceptives present a chemopreventive opportunity for endometrial cancer and ovarian cancer as risk is dramatically lower among women who have used these preparations than among those who have not So, the highest protective effect was produced by preparations with the lowest estrogen and the highest progesterone content. Endometrial cancer risk is not elevated when combined therapy is given in a cyclic manner with progestin administered only part of the time and it is reduced when both oestrogen and progestin are administered on a daily basis (41).In most cases, the endometrioid adenocarcinoma of the endometrium is preceded by hyperplasia with different risk of progression into carcinoma. Two percent of the cases with complex hyperplasia (8/390) progressed into carcinoma and 10.5% into atypical hyperplasia. Fifty-two percent of the atypical hyperplasias (58/112) progressed into carcinomas. In the case of progestogen treatment (n = 208 cases) 61.5% showed remission confirmed by re-curetting, compared with 20.3% of the cases without hormonal treatment (n = 182; $P < 0.0001$). Endometrial hyperplasia without atypia,it is known respond to hormonal treatment. In postmenopausal situation, atypical hyperplasia should be treated with total hysterectomy(42).Endometrial and ovarian cancer are the fourth and fifth most common malignancies in women, with approximately 40,000 new endometrial and 25,000 new ovarian cancers expected to be diagnosed in the Unites States, per year. Combined oral contraceptives reduce the risk of endometrial about 50%. The risk of carcinomas decreases with an increasing duration of oral contraceptive use and this reduced risk lasts for 10-15 years after cessation. A significantly lower risk of developing an endometrial carcinoma can be observed for contraceptives with a high progestin and a low estrogen concentration. Due to the protective effect, the use of oral contraceptives is a useful means chemoprevention in women at high risk of endometrial cancer(43). Although intrauterine progesterone therapy has been proposed as a potential uterine-sparing treatment for atypical endometrial hyperplasia and adenocarcinoma, was reported a case of a woman with atypical endometrial hyperplasia who was treated with the levonorgestrel-releasing intrauterine system for 6 months. At follow-up, she was noted to have an increasing endometrial thickness on ultrasonography, and biopsy revealed progression of her lesion to adenocarcinoma(44). The levonorgestrel-releasing intrauterine system (LNG-IUS) has profound morphologic effects on the endometrium, including gland atrophy and extensive decidual transformation of the stroma. The findings confirm that the stromal compartment of the endometrium undergoes changes consistent with decidualization for at least up to 12 months after insertion of an LNG-IUS. There was no correlation between the study end-points and the menstrual patterns reported by some subjects. Further study of the decidualized nature of the stromal cells in the LNG-exposed endometrium should enhance understanding of the mechanisms responsible for breakthrough bleeding in users of progestogen-only contraceptives.(45).

CERVICAL CANCER RISK

In some studies HCs have been associated with an increased risk of cervical abnormalities and cervical cancer, but there might be alternative explanations for these epidemiological associations: HC users can start having sexual intercourse at an earlier age, they have more sexual partners, and they rarely use barrier methods of contraception(46,47). Nevertheless, combined oral contraceptives are classified by the International Agency for Research on Cancer as a cause of cervical cancer. As the incidence of cervical cancer increases with age, the public-health implications of this association depend largely on the persistence of effects long after use of oral contraceptive has ceased. Among current users of oral contraceptives the risk of invasive cervical cancer increased with increasing duration of use(relative risk= RR for 5 or more years' use versus never use, 1.90)(48).The risk declined after use ceased, and by 10 or more years had returned to that of never users.A similar pattern of risk was seen both for invasive and in-situ cancer, and in women who tested positive for high-risk human papillomavirus(HPV). Relative risk did not vary substantially between women with different characteristics.Ten years' use of oral contraceptives from around age 20 to 30 years is estimated to increase the cumulative incidence of invasive cervical cancer by age 50 from 7.3 to 8.3 per 1000 in less developed countries and, from 3.8 to 4.5 per 1000 in more developed countries (49,50,51). Recent studies suggest that long duration use of oral contraceptives increases the risk of cervical cancer in HPV positive women. Cervical cancer is caused by specific types of the human papilloma virus(HPV)but, not all infected women develop cancer.It was hypothesized that HC can act as a promoter for HPV-induced carcinogenesis (52,53).Available data showed an increase in the transcription of high-risk HPV by the 16alpha–hydroxylation of estrogens and this finding explains the increased cervical carcinogenesis risk for long-term contraceptive using,HPV-infected women (53,54).Results from published studies were combined to examine the relationship between invasive and in situ cervical cancer and duration of use of hormonal contraceptives, with particular attention to HPV infection(55,56). Twenty-eight eligible studies were identified, together including 12.531 women with cervical cancer. Compared with never users of oral contraceptives, the relative risks of cervical cancer increased with increasing duration of use: for durations of approximately less than 5 years, 5-9 years, and 10 or more years, respectively, the summary relative risks were 1.1 , 1.6 , and 2.2 for all women,respectively.The results were similar for invasive and in situ cervical cancers, for squamous cell and adenocarcinoma.(57). The risk was found to increase with use of HCs for more than 7 years beginning after age 25(58).Recently,was affirmed that compared non-users,women who had ever used or currently used HCs had an increased risk of cervical carcinoma.(OR 1.45). However, the risk was not statistically significant.Considering the duration of use, women who had used OC for 3 years or less did not have an increased risk of cervical cancer(OR 0.78).Nevertheless, the odds ratio of oral contraceptive pill use for more than 3 years was 2.57.which was statistically significant. So, long-term use of oral contraceptives might be a cofactor that increases the risk of cervical carcinoma by up to four-fold in women who are positive for cervical HPV(55,56,57). For this reason,many U.S.gynecologists refuse prescription of hormonal contraceptives in women without cervical cancer screening(58). Although the World Health Organization does not recommend any change in oral contraceptive use (59).So,a risk-benefit analysis supports the continuation of contraceptive use among women who have abnormal smears but also, who have access to educational counselling and clinical surveillance(60).Cervical cytological studies reported the significantly high frequency of squamous intraepithelial lesions (SILs) in the early stages of contraception with Norplant insertion, but after 1 year a progressive decline of them was found and ,after 3 years no SIL was seen(61).Data suggest that in adolescents and young women HPV infections and their sequalae,squamous intraepithelial lesions(SILs)occur more commonly among human immunodeficiency(HIV)-infected girls because of the HIVassociated CD4+T-cell immunosuppression(62). However,the risk of developing the HPV-associated precancer high-grade squamous intraepithelial lesion(HSIL)in HIV-infected adolescent is unknown. It seems that the use of hormonal contraceptives,either combined oral contraceptives or intramuscolar MPA ,high cervical mucous concentrations of interleukin-12,a positive HPV test,and a persistent low-grade squamous intraepithelial lesion(LSIL) were significantly associated with the development of HSIL(63).

COLORECTAL CANCER RISK

The association between oral contraceptive use and colorectal cancer have yielded conflicting results.The analysis from a multicenter case-control study, conducted in 6 Italian regions in 1992-96 with data from a 1985-91,yielding a total of 803 women with colon cancer (median age, 61 years), 429 cases of rectal cancer (median age, 62 years), and 2793 controls (median age, 57 years)showed that the protection conferred by oral contraceptives(HC) use was similar when the origin of the neoplasm was in the ascending,transverse,or descending colon. An inverse association was also found between use of HCs and rectal cancer (OR, 0.66), but there was no association with duration of OC use.For colon and rectal cancers combined,a 36% reduction in cancer risk was present among combined oral contraceptive(COC) users(OR,0.64).These findings are consistent with the descriptive epidemiology of colorectal cancer, and experimental findings on estrogen receptors and the colorectal cancer pathway.(64) Other researchers reported that oral contraceptive use showed no significant influence, while users of hormone replacement therapy had a reduced risk of rectal cancer(OR = 0.56).Thus, the association of colorectal cancer with reproductive and menstrual factors is neither strong nor consistent (65) .Similar results were obtained from a large study on 118.404 women which supports as the current or past of oral contraceptives use did not appreciably alter the risk of colorectal cancer(66). Adenomatous polyps (adenomas) are precursors of colorectal cancer.Parity, history of spontaneous or induced abortion, infertility, type of menopause, age at menopause, use of oral contraceptives, and use of menopausal hormone replacement therapy were not associated statistically, with significant adenoma risk, although some possible trends were observed (67). As recognized precursor lesions to colorectal cancer, colorectal adenomatous polyps have been studied to enhance knowledge of colorectal cancer etiology. Although most of the known risk factors for colorectal cancer are also associated with the occurrence of colorectal adenomas; cigarette smoking has had a strong,consistent relationship with colorectal adenomas but is generally not associated with colorectal cancer. The explanation for this paradox is unknown(68) .It is also suggest that the major effect of smoking on the colorectal adenoma-carcinoma sequence occurs in the earlier stages of the formation of adenoma and the development of carcinoma in situ.There is little overall association between colon cancer and oral contraceptive use, parity, age at first birth, hysterectomy or oophorectomy status, or age at menopause. Use of contraceptive hormones at or after age 40,was associated with decreased risk of colon cancer(OR= 0.60), particularly among women with more than five years of use (OR =0.47). While, results from previous studies showed as inconsistent any protective effect against colon cancer. Would be important given the continuing debate over its potential risks and benefits(69). Evidence from epidemiologic studies suggests a possible role of exogenous and endogenous hormones in colorectal carcinogenesis in women.However, with respect to exogenous hormones, in contrast to hormone replacement therapy, few cohort studies have examined oral contraceptive use in relation to colorectal cancer risk. A recent study performed on 88.835 women affirmed that use of oral contraceptives was associated with a modest reduction in the risk of colorectal cancer(OR 0.83).No trend was seen in the ratios with increasing duration of oral contraceptive use .The results are suggestive of an inverse association between oral contraceptive use and colorectal carcinogenesis(70). Previous findings on the associations between oral contraceptive (OC) use and reproductive factors and, risk of colorectal cancer have been inconclusive.Women who had used OCs for 6 months to <3 years had a relative risk of 0.61 relative to never users, with little additional decreased risk being seen with longer duration of use (p for multivariate trend = 0.09). No significant association was observed between reproductive factors and colorectal cancer risk. These findings provide some support for a potential role of HCs in reducing risk of colorectal cancer.(71).These data are consistent with a role for estrogen in altering susceptibility to diet and lifestyle factors possibly, via an insulin-related mechanism.(72). It is hypothesized that estrogen up-regulates insulin-like growth factor(IGF-I) receptors and insuline receptor substrate(IRS-I) levels in the colon, which in turn increases susceptibility to ,obesity-induced, increased levels of insulin. It was further hypothesized that androgens may have similar effects in men given the decline in colon cancer risk associated with BMI with advancing age. The association between body mass index (BMI) and colon cancer has been reported to be different for men and women. Scarce literature has examined if estrogen influences these differences.(73) Epidemiologic and experimental reports suggest that female hormones protect against the development of colorectal cancer, but studies are limited. It was described a case of a patient, in the placebo arm of a 4-year primary chemoprevention trial ,who developed adenomatous polyps and then had eradication of polyps after the administration of oral contraceptives. No change in the prostaglandin levels in the colonic mucosa was noted after polyp elimination, making nonsteroidal anti-inflammatory drug ingestion unlikely as a cause. This report represents the regression of colorectal adenomas with the use of estrogen/progesterone compounds (74).Ever users of oral contraceptives do not benefit from a long-term reduction in colorectal cancer, although current and recent use may confer some protection. Women who have used HRT appear to have important reductions in their risk of colorectal cancer, especially while using these hormones. Further study is needed in order to determine how long any benefits last and whether these are stronger in women exposed to both classes of exogenous hormones(75).

SKIN CANCER RISK

Skin expresses estrogen, progesterone, and androgen receptors. Steroid hormones, such as those contained in oral contraceptives,affect skin cell cycle control.Consequently, they can induce increase of epidermal growth factor signaling, expression of proto-oncogenes, inhibition of apoptosis , DNA replication and, potentially can promote tumor development.However, available evidence suggests that while the skin responds to estrogens, progestins, and androgens, these responses do not significantly increase the risk of developing skin cancer when estrogen exposure is not excessive (76,77).The question of whether oral contraceptives increase the risk for the development of skin cancer,particularly melanoma is still an area of concern(76,77). Several studies confirmed that ever being pregnant,age at first pregnancy, current use of hormonal contraceptives, duration of their use,and age at first use of oral contraceptives have an absence or no consistent association with melanoma(78,79,80). While,women who had had three or more children seem to be significantly protected as compared to nulliparous ones. In fact seems that women with both earlier age at first birth (<20 years) and higher parity(>or=5live birth)have a particular lower risk than women with later age at first birth(>or=25 years) and lower parity.(81,82,83). However, other factors could act ,such as excessive sun exposure.as beach holidays for 3 weeks or more.(82). In fact, history of sunburn and intensive sun-UV exposure,both can are important factors for the development of melanocytic nevi and,indirectly for melanoma(76,83,84). Intermittent and intense sun exposure,during the life, could increase the risk,while prolonged exposure,as during outdoor works,seems not associated with the same risk (85,86).Evidence suggests that there is no causal link between oral contraceptive use and melanoma or with benign melanocytic nevi,nor has a specific subgroup of women been consistently implicated ,as being at increased risk of this disease due to use of oral contraceptives(76,83,84).However, based upon small numbers of cases, there was evidence that changes in nevi during recent pregnancies were a risk factor for melanoma(OR = 2.9)(76,83). Reproductive hormonal factors may have a potential role in cutaneous melanoma but oral contraceptive use does not increase the risk of developing melanoma and generally skin cancer when estrogen exposure is not excessive(86,87,88,89).

Furthermore,women who reported experiencing hyperpigmentation of facial skin during prior pregnancy seem to have a lowered risk for all cutaneous melanoma. Similarly,women who reported use of acne medication(81,89).These aspects should be studied further.These data suggest an overall lack of effect of oral contraceptives on cutaneous melanoma risk, in the women population. Although was evaluated that the relative risk, associated with oral contraceptives use for a long period (5 years or longer),which had begun at least 10 years before the melanoma is 1.5(OR)(86).

Rate of European mortality from cutaneous malignant melanoma(CMM) between 1960 and 1999 have tended to decline since 1990s and this improvement resulted particularly favourable in young women (90).

LIVER CANCER RISK

Liver cell adenomas are rare benign tumors whose incidence has been increasing since 1970(91). They generally occur in otherwise healthy women over age 30 ,who have used hormonal contraceptives (HCs) for five years or longer(92,93). In fact,evidence proved the link between the raise of incidence of hepatic adenomas and the widespread and prolonged use of the"pill" (94,95, 96). Not rarely benign liver tumours are incidental findings on echography. Liver cell adenomas are not premalignant and may undergo reversible change after withdrawal of causative agents,such as oral contraceptives (97,98,99). However, these tumors which regress when OC use stops, can reoccur if HC use is reinstituted or if pregnancy occurs(94,100). The most extensive complication of hepatic adenoma is intratumoral or intraperitoneal hemorrhage, which occurs in 50 to 60 per cent of patients(101).The risk of developing adenoma is increased with duration of oral contraceptive use, and in larger tumors, the hemorrhagic risk is also increased in pill users(93,101).Adenoma also occurs in people with Type Ia glycogen storage disease,and is associated with insulin dependent diabetes(101). Some authors believe that liver cell adenomas are potentially premalignant and could degenerate into hepatocellular carcinoma but there is very few well documented reports of this transformation(101,102,103).Although a recent report shows that 10% of hepatic adenoma progress to hepatocellular carcinoma (102).Really, seems that the transformation might be come from areas of dysplasia in the context of liver cell adenoma. In fact, liver adenoma can regress ,while dysplasia is an irreversible, premalignant change and will eventually progress to hepatocellular carcinoma (104,105,106).It is generally believed that focal nodular hyperplasia(FNH) having a wider age distribution, is not associated with the use of oral contraceptives(107,108). However, a large proportion of women with FNH (50-75%) are HC users, as previous clinical observations affirmed(109). However,in long-term HC users it was emphasized the need of surveillance with ultrasonography.It is known that sex hormones and anabolic – androgenic steroids are implicated in the development and progression of hepatic adenomas. The human liver expresses estrogen and androgen receptors and, experimentally both androgens and estrogens have been implicated in stimulating hepatocyte proliferation and may act as liver tumor inducers or promoters In humans, receptors are present and may mediate the action of sex steroids or androgenic steroids on hepatic adenomas and adiacent liver,but in less than one third of patients.This evidence may have theraepeutic implications(110,111).A paradigmatic case of liver adenoma in a young women affected from Polycystic ovary syndrome associated with high levels of androgen and following a high dose hormonal therapy has been reported(112). So,surveillance can be advised also for women with hormonal imbalance treated with high doses of hormonal therapy.However,the increased risk for hepatocellular carcinoma in the absence of hepatitis B viruses , is the only established evidence of a direct association between HC use and cancer risk,which led an International Agency for Research on Cancer Working Group to classify combined hormonal contraceptives as carcinogenic to humans in 1998(113). The role of estrogens in the genesis of hepatic adenomas is well established, but is more controversial with focal nodular hyperplasia(108, 109). The appearance of low-dose HCs does not seem to have decreased the incidence of benign liver tumors.Therefore, several studies have demonstrated that the risk of adenoma increase with the duration of treatment. In the mean time.benign liver tumors are very rare and should not affect prescription of HCs. Focal nodular hyperplasia of liver is less dangerous than hepatic adenomas but still necessitate stopping use.This pathological entity had been reported in women prior to widespread use of the pill,but HCs use appear to favor its growth. Some cases of subhepatic vein thrombosis or the Budd-Chiari syndrome, associated to focal nodular hyperplasia as well as adenoma have been reported (114, 115,116).

OTHER CANCER RISKS

Neurofibromas growth

Neurofibromas are benign tumors of the peripheral nerve sheath, which may occur sporadically and, in association with the common familial cancer syndrome, neurofibromatosis type 1(NF 1).NF1 is a hereditary disease caused by mutations of the NF1 gene at 17q11.2. Loss of the NF1 gene product in Schwann cells leads to the development of benign nerve sheath tumors(117).There are intriguing links between the growth of neurofibromas and levels of circulating hormones: in fact, dermal neurofibromas usually arise during puberty, increase in number and size during pregnancy, and shrink after giving birth. The majority (75%) of neurofibromas express progesterone receptor(PR), whereas only a minority (5%) of neurofibromas express estrogen receptor(ER).It has been suggested that hormones may influence the neurofibromas of patients with NF1 and may increase potential for malignant transformation of plexiform tumors. Within neurofibromas, PR is expressed by non-neoplastic tumor-associated cells and not by neoplastic Schwann cells. We hypothesize that progesterone may play an important role in neurofibroma growth and suggest that antiprogestins may be useful in the treatment of this tumor.(118,119,120).

Pancreatic cancer risk

Incidence rates for pancreatic cancer are consistently lower in women than in men. Previous studies suggested that reproductive factors, particularly parity, may reduce pancreatic cancer risk in women. During a study on 115,474 women(follow-up: 22 years), 243 cases of pancreatic cancer were identified. Compared with nulliparous women, the relative risk of pancreatic cancer was 0.86 for women with 1-2 births, 0.75 for 3-4 births, and 0.58 for those with 5 or more births ,after adjusting for other factors. The analysis for linear trend indicated a 10% reduction in risk for each birth.Other reproductive factors and exogenous hormone use were not significantly, related to pancreatic cancer risk(121). Compared with women who were premenopausal at baseline, postmenopausal women were at significantly increased risk of pancreatic cancer (odds ratio = 2.44) Age at first live birth, parity, age at menarche, use of oral contraceptive, and use of hormone replacement therapy (HRT) were not associated with altered pancreatic cancer risk in studies population. However, among parous women, later age at first full-term pregnancy ,significantly increases the risk of this cancer (adjusted OR = 4.05).Other than the increased risk among postmenopausal women, this cohort study provides little support for associations with hormonal factors. Additional prospective data are needed. However, growing epidemiological evidence that aspects of reproductive history and hormonal exposure are associated with risk of this disease could induce to support the hypothesis that pancreatic cancer is, at least in part, an estrogen-dependent disease

(122). Prolonged lactation and increased parity seem associated with a reduced risk for pancreatic cancer(123) In a parallel fashion, risk of pancreatic cancer was decreased for women with intact ovaries compared to those who had oophorectomy: hazard ratio was 0.70.These results indicate that older age at menopause are associated with reduced pancreatic cancer risk, but further research is warranted.(124). It was observed no association between any other reproductive factors examined (age at first birth, menarche, or menopause; type of menopause; diethylstilbestrol (DES) use; or duration of oral contraceptive or estrogen replacement therapy use) and pancreatic cancer mortality(125). In summary, literature data support the observation that high parity is associated with lower risk of pancreatic cancer but do not show a linear trend with increasing parity. Furthermore, we find no evidence that other reproductive factors are associated with pancreatic cancer mortality.(126). It is of interest to report that clinically attainable concentrations of Medroxyprogesterone acetate (MPA) can inhibit the growth of some human pancreatic carcinoma cells, in vitro, by inducing apoptosis, probably through their PR, in association with the phosphorylation of bcl-2 (127).

Unclear cancer risks

Literature data no reported significant association of age at menarche, parity, age at first birth, and exogenous hormone use with bladder cancer risk. Findings suggest that menopausal status and age at menopause may play a role in modifying bladder cancer risk among women (128). For postmenopausal women, early age at menopause (</=45 years) compared with late age at menopause (>/=50 years) was reported associated with a statistically significant increased risk of bladder cancer (incidence rate ratio = 1.63). The association between age at menopause and bladder cancer risk could be modified by cigarette smoking status(1,129). Greater incidence of thyroid cancer in women than men, particularly evident during the reproductive years, has led to the suggestion that female hormones may increase the risk for this disease.A study estimating the relative risk of papillary thyroid cancer among users of exogenous hormones among 410 women aged 45 to 64 years, observed no association of use of ormonal contraceptives (HCs) or HRT with risk of papillary thyroid cancer. Among women less than 45 years of age, risk of papillary thyroid cancer was reduced in women who had ever used HCs (OR = 0.6); beyond the relation with ever-use, there was no further association with specific aspects of exposure such as estrogenic potency, latency, recency, age at first or last use, or use at the reference date. Therfore, the data do not support the hypothesis that use of exogenous estrogens increases the risk of female thyroid cancer(130).The role of exogenous hormone exposures in the development of meningioma is unclear. Little evidence of associations between meningioma and exogenous hormone exposures in women was found but did suggest that some hormonal exposures may influence tumor biology in those women who develop meningioma(131).

REFERENCES

[1] La Vecchiam, C., Negri, E., Franceschi, S., Parazzini, F. (1993). Long-term impact of reproductive factors on cancer risk. *Int J Cancer*, Jan 21, 53(2), 215-9.

[2] Medard, M.L., Ostrowska, L. (2007).Combined oral contraception and the risk of reproductive organs cancer in women .*Ginekol Pol*, Aug,78(8), 637-41.

[3] Casey, P.M., Cerhan, J.R., Pruthi, S. (2008).Oral contraceptive use and risk of breast cancer. *Mayo Clin Proc*,Jan,83),86-90

[4] Deligeoroglou, E., Michailidis, E., Creatsas, G. (2003).Oral contraceptives and reproductive system cancer. *Ann N Y Acad Sci*,Nov,997,199-208.

[5] White, E., Malone, K.E., Weiss, N.S., Daling, J.R. (1994).Breast cancer among young US women in relation to oral contraceptive use. *J. Nati Cancer Inst*, 86(7), 505-14

[6] Brohet, R.M., Goldgar, D.E., Easton, D.F., Antoniou, A.C., Andrieu, N., Chang-Claude, J., Peock, S., Eeles, R.A., Cook, M., Chu, C., Noguès, C., Lasset, C., Berthet, P., Meijers-Heijboer, H., Gerdes, A.M., Olsson, H., Caldes, T., van Leeuwen, F.E., Rookus, M.A. (2007).Oral contraceptives and breast cancer risk in the international BRCA1/2 carrier cohort study: a report from EMBRACE, GENEPSO, GEO-HEBON, and the IBCCS Collaborating Group.*J Clin Oncol*, Sep 1,25(25), 3831-6.

[7] Haile, R.W.,Thoma, D.C., McGuire, V., Felberg, A., John, E.M., Milne, R.L., Hopper, J.L. et.al. (2006).BRCA1 and BRCA2 mutation carriers,oral contraceptives use,and breast cancer before age 50. *Cancer Epidemiol.Biomarker Prev*, 15(10),1863-70.

[8] Daling, J.R., Brinton, L.A., Voigt, L.F., Weiss, N.S., Coates, R.J., Malone, K.E., Schoenberg, J.B., Gammon, M. (1996). Risk of breast cancer among white women following induced abortion. *Am J Epidemiol*,Aug 15,144(4), 373-80.

[9] Daling, J.R., Malone, K.E., Voigt, L.F., White, E., Weiss, N.S. (1997).Risk of breast cancer among young women: relationship Med to induced abortion.*N Engl J*, 336(2), 81-5

[10] Rookus, M.A., van Leeuwen, F.E. (1996).Induced abortion and risk for breast cancer: reporting (recall) bias in a Dutch case-control study. *J Natl Cancer Inst*, 88 (23),1759-64

[11] Van Leeuwen, F.E. (1991).Epidemiologic aspects of exogenous progestagens in relation to their role in pathogenesis of human breast cancer. *Acta Endocrinol*, 125(1), 13.

[12] Kodama, M., Kodama, T., Seeger, H., Rakov, V., Mueck, A.O. (1981).Adolescence, a critical stage for the genesis of female cancers (review)*Anticancer Res*,1(2), 93-9.

[13] La Vecchia, C.,Tavani, A., Franceschi, S., Parazzini, F. (1996).Oral contraceptives and cancer.A review of the evidence.*Drug Saf*, 14(4), 260-72.

[14] Seeger, H., Rakov, V., Mueck, A.O. (2005). Dose-dependent changes of the ratio of apoptosis to proliferation by norethisterone and medroxyprogesterone acetate in human breast epithelial cells. *Horm Metab Res*,Aug, 37(8), 468-73.

[15] Sweeney, C., Giuliano, A.R., Baumgartner, K.B., Byers, T., Herrick, J.S., Edwards, S.L., Slattery, M.L. (2007).Oral ,injected and implanted contraceptives and breat cancer risk among US Hispanic and non-Hispanic white women. *Int. J. Cancer*,121 (11), 2517-23.

[16] Altaha, R., Reed, E., Abraham, J.Breast and ovarian cancer genetics and prevention.)Burke, W., Daly, M., Garber, J., Botkin, M.J., Lynch, P., McTiernan, A., Offit, K. (2003). *WV Med J*,99(5),187-91.

[17] Fraser, I.S., Kovacs, G.T. (2003). The efficacy of non-contraceptive uses for hormonal contraceptives. *Med J Aust,* Jun 16,178(12),621-3.

[18] Kehoe, S.M., Kauff, N.D. (2007).Screening and prevention of hereditary gynecologic cancers. *Semin Oncol*,Oct, 34(5), 406-10.

[19] Burke, W., Daly, M., Garber, J., Botkin, M.J., Lynch, P., McTiernan, A., Offit, K., Periman, J., Petersen, G.,Thomson, E.,Varricchio,C. Recommendations for follow-up care of individuals with an inherited predisposition to cancer. II BRCA1 and BRCA2. Cancer Genetics Studies Consortiun. *JAMA,*26, 277(12),997-1003. Review.

[20] Verheijen, R.H., Boonstra, H., Menko, F.H., de Graaff, J., Vasen, H.F., Kenter, G.G. (2002). Recommendations for the management of women with an increased genetic risk of gynaecological cancer. *Ned Tijdschr Geneeskd*, Dec 14,146(50), 2414-8.

[21] Casey, M.J., Synder, C., Bewtra, C., Narod, S.A., Watson, P., Lynch, H.T. (2005).Intra- abdominal carcinomatosis after prophylactic oophorectomy in women of hereditary breast ovarian cancer syndrome associated with BRCA1 and BRCA2 mutations. *Gynecol Oncol*,May, 97(2), 457-67.
[22] Merki-Feld, G.S., Seeger, H., Mueck, A.O. (2008).Comparison of the proliferative effects of ethinylestradiol on human breast cancer cells in an intermittent and a continuous dosing regime. *Horm Metab Res*, Mar, 40(3), 206-9.
[23] Krämer, E.A., Seeger, H., Krämer, B., Wallwiener, D., Mueck, A.O. (2006).The effect of progesterone, testosterone and synthetic progestogens on growth factor- and estradiol-treated human cancerous and benign breast cells.*Eur J Obstet Gynecol Reprod Biol*, Nov,129(1), 77-83.
[24] Hanna, L., Adams, M. (2006).Prevention of ovarian cancer.*Best Pract. Res. Obstet.Gynaecol*, 20(2), 339-627.
[25] Persson, I. (2000). Estrogens in the causation of breast, endometrial and ovarian cancers – evidence and hypotheses from epidemiological findings. *J Steroid Biochem Mol Biol*, 74(5), 357-64.
[26] Riman, T., Nilsson, S., Persson, I.R. (2004). Review of epidemiological evidence for reproductive and hormonal factors in relation to the risk of epithelial ovarian malignancies. *Acta Obstet. Gynecol. Scand*, 83(9),783-95
[27] Greer, J.B., Modugno, F., Allen, G.O., Auranen, A., Hietanen, S., Salmi, T.,Grénman, S. (2005). Hormonal treatments and epithelial ovarian cancer risk. *Int. J. Gynaecol Cancer*,15(5), 692-700.
[28] Burkman RT. (2002).Reproductive hormones and cancer: ovarian and colon cancer. *Obstet Gynecol Clin North Am*, Sep,29(3), 527-40.
[29] Beral, V., Doll, R., Hermon, C., Peto, R., Reeves, G. (2008).Collaborative Group on Epidemiological Studies of Ovarian Cancer. Ovarian cancer and oral contraceptives:collaborative reanalysis of data from 45 epidemiological studies including 23,257 women with ovarian cancer and 87,303 controls. *Lancet*, Jan 26, 371(9609), 303-14.
[30] Ness, R.B. (2005). Androgenic progestins in oral contraceptives and the risk of epithelial ovarian cancer. *Obstet. Gynecol*, 105(4), 731-40.
[31] Sanderson, M.,Williams, M.A.,Weiss, N.S., Hendrix, N,W., Chauhan, S.P. (2006).Oral contraceptives and epithelial ovarian cancer.Does dose matter? *J.Reprod.Med*,45(9), 720-6.
[32] Lurie, G.,Thompson, P., McDuffie, K.E., Carney, M.E.,Terada, K.Y.,Goodman, M.T. (2007). Association of estrogen and progestin potency of oral contraceptives with ovarian carcinoma risk. *Obstet.Gynecol*,109(3), 597-607.

[33] Schildkraut, J.M.,Calingaert, B.,Manchbanks, P.A., Moorman, P.G., Rodriguez, G.C. (2002). Impact of progestin and estrogen potency in oral contraceptives on ovarian cancer risk. *J.Natl.Cancer*, 94(1), 32-8.

[34] Lancaster, J.M., Powell, C.B., Kauff, N.D., Cass, I., Chen, L.M., Lu, K.H., Mutch, D.G.,Berchuck, A., Karlan, B.Y., Herzog, T.J. (2007).Society of Gynecologic Oncologists Education Committee.Society of Gynecologic Oncologists Education Committee statement on risk assessment for inherited gynecologic cancer predispositions. *Gynecol Oncol,*107 (2), 159-62.

[35] Pujol P,This P,Noruzinia M,Stoppa –Lyonnet D,Maudelonde T. (2004). Are the hereditary forms of BRCA 1 and BRCA 2 breast cancer sensitive to estrogens? *Bull.Cancer*, 91(7-8),583 91.

[36] Auranen, A., Hietanen, S., Salmi, T., Grénman, S. Hormonal treatments and epithelial ovarian cancer risk. *Int J Gynecol Cancer*, 15(5), 692-700. 35)

[37] The ESHRE Capri Workshop Group. Noncontraceptive health benefits of combined oral contraception. (2005). *Hum. Reprod. Update*, 11(5), 513-25

[38] Pike, M.C., Spicer, D.V. (2000). Hormonal contraception and chemoprevention of female cancers. *Endocr Relat Cancer*, Jun, 7(2), 73-83.

[39] Henderson, B.E., Ross, R.K., Pike, M.C. (1993). Hormonal chemoprevention of cancer in women. *Science*, 259(5095),633-8.

[40] Maxwell, G.L., Schildkraut, J.M., Calingaert, B., Risinger, J.I., Dainty, L., Marchbanks, P.A., Berchuck, A., Barrett, J.C., Rodriguez, G.C. (2006). Progestin and estrogen potency of combination oral contraceptives and endometrial cancer risk. *Gynecol Oncol*, Nov,103(2), 535-40.

[41] Voight, L.F., Deng, Q.,Wwiss, N.S. (1994). Recency,duration,and progestin content of oral contraceptives in relation to the incidence of endometrial cancer.*Cancer Causes.Control*,5(3), 227-33.

[42] Bernstein, L. (2006). The risk of breast, endometrial and ovarian cancer in users of hormonal preparations. *Basic Clin Pharmacol Toxicol*, Mar, 98(3), 288-96

[43] Horn, L.C., Schnurrbusch, U., Bilek, K., Hentschel, B., Einenkel, J. (2004). Risk of progression in complex and atypical endometrial hyperplasia: clinicopathologic analysis in cases with and without progestogen treatment. *Int J Gynecol Cancer*,14(2),348-53.

[44] Medl, M. (1998).Oral contraceptives and endometrial and ovarian carcinomas.*Gynakol Geburtshilfliche Rundsch*, 38(2), 105-8.

[45] Kresowik, J., Ryan, G.L., Van Voorhis, B.J. (2008). Progression of atypical endometrial hyperplasia to adenocarcinoma despite intrauterine

progesterone treatment with the levonorgestrel-releasing intrauterine system. *Obstet Gynecol*,111(2), 547- 9.
[46] Rizkalla, H.F., Higgins, M., Kelehan, P., O'Herlihy, C. (2008). Pathological findings associated with the presence of a mirena intrauterine system at hysterectomy.*Int J Gynecol Pathol*, Jan, 27(1),74-8.
[47] Prilepskala, V.N., Kondrikov, N.I., Nazarova, N.M. (1991). Morphofunctional features of the cervix uteri in women using hormonal contraception Akush.*Ginekol.(Mosk),*12, 6-10.
[48] International Collaboration of Epidemiological Studies of Cervical Cancer. Appleby, P., Beral, V., Berrington de González, A., Colin, D., Franceschi, S., Goodhill, A., Green, J., Peto, J., Plummer, M., Sweetland, S. (2007). Cervical cancer and hormonal contraceptives: collaborative reanalysis of individual data for 16,573 women with cervical cancer and 35,509 women without cervical cancer from 24 epidemiological studies.*Lancet*, 370(9599), 1609-21.
[49] Shapiro, S., Rosenberg, L., Hoffman, M., Kelly, J.P.,Cooper, D.D.,Carrara, H., Denny, L.E., du Toit, G., Allan, B.R.,Stander, I.A.,Williamson, A.L. (2003). Risk of invasive cancer of the cervix in relation to the use of injectable progestogen contraceptives and combined estrogen/progestogen oral contraceptives. *Cancer Causes Control*, 14(5), 485-95.
[50] Syrjanen, K., Shabalova, I., Petrovichev, N., Kozachenko, V., Zakharova, T., Pajanidi, J., Podistov, J., Chemeris, G., Sozaeva, L., Lipova, E.,Tsidaeva, I. (2006). Oral contraceptives are not an independent risk factor for cervical intraepithelial neoplasia or high-risk human papillomavirus infections. *Anticancer Res*,26(6C),4729-40.
[51] De Villiers, E.M. (2003).Relationship between steroid hormone contraceptives and HPV, cervical intraepithelial neoplasia and cervical carcinoma.*Int.J.Cancer*, 103(6), 70
[52] Moodley, M., Moodley, J.,Chetty, R., Herrington, C.S. (2003). The role of steroid contraceptive hormones in the pathogenesis of invasive cervical cancer:a review. *Int.J.Gynecol.Cancer*, 13(2), 103-10
[53] Green, J., Berrington deGonzales, A., Smith, J.S.M., Franceschi, S., Appleby, P., Plummer, M., Beral, V. (2003). Human papillomavirus and use of oral contraceptives.*Br.J.Cancer*,88(11),1713-20.
[54] Smith, J.S., Green, J., Berrington de Gonzalez, A., Appleby, P., Peto, J., Plummer, M., Franceschi,S., Beral, V. (2003). Cervical cancer and use of hormonal contraceptives: a systematic review. *Lancet*, Apr 5, 361(9364), 1159-67.

[55] Le, M.G., Bachelot, A., Doyen, F., Kramar, A. (1985). A study on the association between the use of oral contraception and cancer of the breast or cervix:preliminary findings of a French study. *Contracept.Fertil.Sex(Paris)*, 13(3), 553-8.
[56] Vanakankovit N.,Taneepanichskul S. (2008). Effect of oral contraceptives on risk of cervical cancer. *J.Med.Assoc. Thai*, 91(1), 7-12.
[57] Moreno, V., Bosch, F.X., Munoz, N., Meijer, C.J., Shah, K.V.,Walboomers, J.M., Herrero, R., Franceschi, S. (2002). International Agency for Research on Cancer,Multicentric Cervical Cancer Study Group. Effect of oral contraceptives on risk of cervical cancer in women with human papillomavirus infection:the IARC multicentric case-control study. *Lancet*, 359 (9312), 1085-92.
[58] Sasieni, P. (2007). Cervical cancer prevention and hormonal contraception. *Lancet*,370 (9599),1591-2.
[59] Scharz, E.B., Saint, M.,Gildengorin, G.,Weitz,T.A., Stewart, F.H., Sawaya, G.F. (2005).Cervical cancer screening continues to limit provision of contraception. *Contraception*, 72(3), 179-81.
[60] Bertram, C.C. (2004). Evidence for practice:oral contraception and risk of cervical cancer. *J. Am. Acad.Nurse Pract*, 16(10),455-61.
[61] Misra, J.S.,Tandon, P.,Srivastava, A.,Das, K., Chandrawati Saxena, N.C. (2003). Cervical cytological studies in women inserted with Norplant-contraceptive.*Diagn.Cytopathol*,29(3), 136-9.
[62] Moscicki, A.B., Ellenberg, J.H.,Vermund, S.H., Holland, C.A., Darragh, T., Crowley-Nowick, P.A., Levin, L.,Wilson, C.M. (2000).Prevalence of and risks for cervical human papillomavirus infection and squamous intraepithelial lesions in adolescent girls:impact of infection with human immunodeficiency virus.*Arch.Pediatr.Adolesc.Med*, 154(2), 127-34.
[63] Moscicki, A.B., Ellenberg, J.H., Crowley-Nowick, P., Darragh, T.M., Xu, J., Fahrat, S, (2004). Risk of high-grade squamous intraepithelial lesion in HIV-infected adolescents.*J.Infect.Dis*, 190(8),1413-21
[64] Fernandez, E., La Vecchia, C., Franceschi, S., Braga, C., Talamini, R., Negri, E., Parazzini, F. (1998). Oral contraceptive use and risk of colorectal cancer. *Epidemiology*,9(3), 295-300.
[65] Talamini, R., Franceschi, S., Dal Maso, L., Negri, E., Conti, E., Filiberti, R., Montella, M., Nanni, O., La Vecchia, C. (1998).The influence of reproductive and hormonal factors on the risk of colon and rectal cancer in women. *Eur J Cancer*, 34(7), 1070-6.
[66] Chute, C.G., Willett, W.C., Colditz, G.A., Stampfer, M.J., Rosner, B., Speizer, F.E. (1991).A prospectivestudy of reproductive history and

exogenous estrogens on the risk of colorectal cancer in women.*Epidemiology*, May, 2(3), 201-7.
[67] Jacobson, J.S., Neugut, A.I., Garbowski, G.C., Ahsan, H., Waye, J.D.,Treat, M.R., Forde, K.A. (1995). Reproductive risk factors for colorectal adenomatous polyps (New York City, NY, United States). *Cancer Causes Control*, Nov, 6(6), 513-8.
[68] Potter, J.D., Bigler, J., Fosdick, L., Bostick, R.M., Kampman, E., Chen, C., Louis, T.A., Grambsch, P. (1999).Colorectal adenomatous and hyperplastic polyps: smoking and N-acetyltransferase 2 polymorphisms.*Cancer Epidemiol Biomarkers Prev*, 8(1), 69-75.
[69] Jacobs, E.J., White, E., Weiss, N.S. (1994). Exogenous hormones, reproductive history, and colon cancer (Seattle, Washington, USA). *Cancer Causes Control*,Jul, 5(4), 359-66
[70] Kabat, G.C., Miller, A.B., Rohan, T.E. (2008).Oral contraceptive use, hormone replacement therapy, reproductive history and risk of colorectal cancer in women. *Int J Cancer*, 1,122(3), 643-6.
[71] Lin, J., Zhang, S.M., Cook, N.R., Manson, J.E., Buring, J.E., Lee, I.M. (2007). Oral contraceptives, reproductive factors, and risk of colorectal cancer among women in a prospective cohort study. *Am J Epidemiol*, 165(7), 794-801.
[72] Slattery, M.L., Ballard-Barbash, R., Potter, J.D., Ma, K.N., Caan, B.J., Anderson, K., Samowitz, W. (2004).Sex-specific differences in colon cancer associated with p53 mutations.*Nutr Cancer*,49(1), 41-8.
[73] Slattery, M.L., Ballard-Barbash, R., Edwards, S., Caan, B.J., Potter, J.D. (2003). Body mass index and colon cancer: an evaluation of the modifying effects of estrogen (United States).*Cancer Causes Control*, 14(1), 75-84.
[74] Giardiello, F.M., Hylind, L.M., Trimbath, J.D., Hamilton, S.R., Romans, K.E., Cruz-Correa, M., Corretti, M.C., Offerhaus, G.J., Yang, V.W. (2005).Oral contraceptives and polyp regression in familial adenomatous polyposis. *Gastroenterology*, Apr,128(4), 1077-80.
[75] Hannaford, P., Elliott, A.1. (2005).Use of exogenous hormones by women and colorectal cancer: evidence from the Royal College of General Practitioners' Oral Contraception Study. *Contraception*,71(2), 95-8.
[76] Leslie, K.K., Espey, E. (2005).Oral contraceptives and skin cancer:is there a link? *Am.J.Clin. Dermatol*, 6(6), 349-55.
[77] Piérard, G.E.,Piérard –Franchimont, C.,Quatresooz, P., Kridelka, F.,Gaspard, U. (2007).Groupe Mosan d'Etudes Tumeurs Pigmentaires. Can we sort out from the jumble about oral contraceptives and skin cancer? *Rev.Med.Liege*, 62(5-6),463-6.

[78] Gefeller, O., Hassan, K.,Wille, L. (1988).Cutaneous malignant melanoma in women and the role of oral contraceptives. *Br.J.Dermatol*, 138(1), 122-4.
[79] Lea, C.S., Holly, E.A., Hartge, P., Lee, J.S., Guerry, D. (2007). 4th ,Elder DE,Halpern A,Sagebiel RW, Tucker MA. Reproductive risk factors for cutaneous melanoma in women:a case- control study.*Am.J.Epidemiol*, 165(5), 505-13.
[80] Smith, M.A., Fine, J.A., Barnhill, R.L., Berwick, M. (1998). Hormonal and reproductive influences and risk of melanoma in women. *Int.j.Epidemiol*, 27(5), 751-7.
[81] Holly, E.A.,Cress, R.D., Ahn, D.K. (1995).Cutaneous melanoma in women.III.Reproductive factors and oral contraceptive use. *Am.J.Epidemiol*, 141(10), 943-50.
[82] Naldi, L.,Altieri, A., Imberti, G.E.,Giordano, L.,Gallus, S., LaVecchia, C. (2005). Oncology Study Group of the Italian Group for Epidemiologic Research in Dermatology(GISED). Cutaneous malignant melanoma in women.Phenotypic characteristics,sun exposure, and hormonal factors:a case control study from Italy.*Ann.Epidemiol*,15(7), 545-50.
[83] Osterlind, A. (1992).Hormonal and reproductive factors in melanoma risk.*Clin.Dermatol*,10(1), 75-8.
[84] Zanetti, R., Franceschi, S., Rosso, S., Bidoli, E.,Colonna, S. (1990).Cutaneous malignant melanoma in females:the role of hormonal and reproductive factors.*Int.J. Epidemiol*,19(3),522-6.
[85] Breitbart, M.,Garbe, C., Buttner P,Weiss, J., Soyer, H.P., Stocker, U., Kruger, S., Breitbart, E.W., Weckbecker, J., Panizzon, R., Bahmer, F., Tilgen, W., Guggenmoos-Holzmann, I., Orfanos, C.E. (1997).Ultraviolet light exposure ,pigmentary traits and the development of melanocytic naevi and cutaneous melanoma.A case-control study of the German Central Malignant Melanoma Registry. *Acta Derm.Venereol*, 77(5), 374-8.
[86] Beral, V., Evans, S., Shaw, H., Milton, G. (1984). Oral contraceptive use and malignant melanoma in Australia. *Br.J.Cancer*, 50(5), 681-5.
[87] Karagas, M.R., Zens, M.S., Stukel, T.A., Swerdiow, A.J., Rosso, S., Osterlind, A., Mack, T., Kirkpatrick, C., Holly, E.A., Green, A., Gallagher, R., Elwood, J.M., Armstrong, B.K. (2006). Pregnancy history and incidence of melanoma in women:a pooled analysis.*Cancer Causes Control*,17(1), 11-9.
[88] Green, A. (1991). Oral contraceptives and skin neoplasia.*Contraception*, 43(6), 653-66.

[89] Rosso, S., Zanetti, R., Pippione, M., Sancho-Garnier, H. (1998).Parallel risk assessment of melanoma and basal cell carcinoma :skin characteristics and sun exposure. *Melanoma Res*, 8(6), 573-83.
[90] Bosetti C,La Vecchia C,Naldi L,Lucchini F,Negri E,Levi F. (2004).Mortality from cutaneous malignant melanoma in Europe.Has the epidemic level off? *Melanoma Res*,14(4), 301-9.
[91] Nissen, E.D., Kent, D.R., Nissen, S.E. (1979).Role of oral contraceptive agents in the pathogenesis of liver tumors. *J Toxicol Environ Health*,5(2-3),231-54.
[92] Ruiz Lòpez, D., Sànchez Salvador, J., Fèrnandez Martin, C., Anton Diaz, E. (2005). Hepatic adenoma related to oral contraceptives use. *Aten.Primaria*,35(2), 109-10.
[93] Ferrara, B.E., Rutland, E.D. (1988).Liver tumor in long-term user of oral contraceptives. *Postgrad. Med*, 84(6), 107-9.
[94] Teeuwen, P.H., Ruers, T.J.,Wobbes, T. (2007). Hepatocellular adenoma,a tumour particularly seen in mostly young women. Ned.Tijdschr.Geneeeskd. 151(24),1321-4.
[95] Barthelmes, L.,Tait, I.S. (2005). Liver cell adenoma and liver cell adenomatosis.*HPB (Oxford)*,7(3), 186-96.
[96] Sherlock, S. (1979).Hepatic adenomas and oral contraceptives. *J.Toxicol. Environ.Health*, 5(3), 231-54.
[97] Aseni, P., Sansalone, C.V., Sammartino, C., Benedetto, F.D., Carrfiello, G., Giacomoni, A.,Osio, C., Vertemati, M., Forti, D. (2001). Rapid disappearance of hepatic adenoma after contraceptive withdrawal. *J.Clin.Gastroenterol*, 33(3), 234-6.
[98] Steinbrecher,V.P., Lisbona, R., Huang, S.N.,Mishkin, S. (1981). Complete regression of hepatocellular adenoma after withdrawal of oral contraceptives.*Dig.Dis.Sci*,26(11),1045-50.
[99] Svrcek, M., Jeannot, E., Arrivè, L., Poupon, R., Fromont, G., Flèjou, J.F., Zucman-Rossi, J., Bouchard, P., Wendum, D. (2007). Regressive liver adenomatosis following androgenic progestin therapy withdrawal: a case report with a 10-year follow-up and a molecular analysis. *Uur.J. Endocrinol*, 156(6), 617-21.
[100] Gordon, S.C., Reddy, K.R., Livingstone, A.S., Jeffers, L.J. (1986).Schiff ERResolution of a contraceptive- steroid-induced hepatic adenoma with subsequent evolution into hepatocellular carcinoma.*Ann. Intern.Med*, 105(4), 547-9

[101] Ito, M., Sasaki, M.,Wen, C.Y., Nakashima, M.,Ueki, T., Ishibashi, H.,Yano, M., Kage, M. (2003). Liver cell adenoma with malignant transformation: a case report. *World J.Gastroenterol,*9 (10), 2379-81.
[102] Gyorffy, E.J., Bredfeldt, J.E., Black, W.C. (1989). Transformation of hepatic cell adenoma to hepatocellular carcinoma due to oral contraceptive use.*Ann.Intern.Med*, 110(6), 489-90
[103] Herman, P., Machado, M.A.,Volpe, P., Pugliese, V.,Vianna, M.R., Bacchella, T., Machado, M.C., Pinotti, H.W. (1994). Transformation of hepatic adenoma into hepatocellular carcinoma in patients with prolonged use of oral contraceptives. *Rev.Hosp.Clin.Fac.Med.Sao Paulo*, 49(1), 30-3.
[104] Korula, J.,Yellin, A.,Kanel, G.,Campofiori, G., Nichols, P. (1991). Hepatocellular carcinoma coexisting with hepatic adenoma.Incidental discovery after long-term oral contraceptive use.*West J.Med*, 155(4), 416-8 .
[105] Perret, A.G., Mosnier, J.F., Porcheron, J.,Cuilleron, M., Berthoux, P.,Boucheron, S., Audigier, J.C. (1996). Role of oral contraceptives in the growth of a multilobular adenoma associated with a hepatocellular carcinoma in a young woman. *J.Hepatol*, 25(6), 976-9.
[106] Tao, L.C. (1991). Oral contraceptives-associated liver cell adenoma and hepatocellular carcinoma.Cytomorphology and mechanism of malignant transformation. *Cancer,* 68(2), 341-7.
[107] Shortell, C.K., Schwartz, S.I. (1991).Hepatic adenoma and focal nodular hyperplasia.*Surg. Gynecol.Obstet*, 173(5), 426-31.
[108] Tajada, M., Nerin, J., Ruiz, M.M., Sanchez-Dehesa, M., Fabre, E. (2001).Liver adenoma and focal nodular hyperplasia associated with oral contraceptives.*Eur.J.Contracept.Reprod.Health Care*, 6(4),227-30.
[109] Scalori, A.,Tafani, A.,Gallus, S., La Vecchia, C., Colombo, M. (2002). Oral contraceptives and the risk of focal nodular hyperplasia of the liver:a case – control study. *Am.J.Obstet. Gynecol*, 186(2), 195-7.
[110] Giannitrapani, L., Soresi, M., La Spada, E., Cervello, M., D'Alessandro, N., Montalto, G. (2006). Sex hormones and risk of liver tumor. *Ann N Y Acad Sci*,1089,228-36
[111] Torbenson, M., Lee, J.H., Choti, M., Gage, W., Abraham, S.C., Montgomery, E., Boitnott, J., Wu, T.T. (2002). Hepatic adenomas: analysis of sex steroid receptor status and the Wnt signaling pathway. *Mod Pathol*, 15(3),189-96
[112] Cohen, C., Lawson, D., DeRose, P.B. (1998).Sex and androgenic steroid receptor expression in hepatic adenomas.*Hum.Pathol*, 29(12), 1428-32.Toso, C., Rubbia –Brandt, L., Negro, F., Morel, P., Mentha, G. (2003).

Hepatocellular adenoma and polycystic ovary syndrome.*Liver Int*,23(1), 35-7.
[113] La Vecchia, C., Altieri, A., Franceschi, S., Tavani, A. (2001).Oral contraceptives and cancer: an update.*Drug Saf*, 24(10), 741-54.
[114] Shilling, M.K., Zimmermann, A., Radaelli, C., Seiler, C.A., Buchler, M.W. (2000).Liver nodules resembling focal nodular hyperplasia after hepatic venous thrombosis.*J.Hepatol*, 33(4), 673-6.
[115] Tong, H.K., Fai, G.L., Ann, L.T., Hock, O.B. (1981). Budd-Chiari syndrome and hepatic adenomas associated with oral contraceptives.A case report. *Singapore Med.J*, 22(3), 168-72.
[116] Buhler, H., Pirovino, M., Akoblantz, A., Altofer, J., Weitzel, M., Maranta, E., Schmid, M. (1982). Regression of liver cell adenoma.A follow-up study of three consecutive patients after discontinuation of oral contraceptive use.*Gastroenterology*, 82(4), 775-82.
[117] Overdiek, A.,Winner, U., Mayatepek, E., Rosenbaum, T. (2008).Schwann cells from human neurofibromas show increased proliferation rates under the influence of progesterone. *Pediatric.Res*, Mar 19 (Epub ahead of print).
[118] McLaughlin, M.E., Jacks, T. (2003).Progesterone receptor expression in neurofibromas.*Cancer Res*, 63(4), 752-5.
[119] Fishbein, L., Zhang, X., Fisher, L.B., Li, H., Campbell-Thompson, M.,Yachnis, A., Rubenstein, A., Muir, D.,Wallace, M.R. (2007). In vitro studies of hormones in neurofibromtosis 1 and Schwann cells. *Mol.Carcinog*, 46(7), 512-23.
[120] Lammert, M., Mautner, V.F., Kluwe, L. (2005). Do hormonal contraceptives stimulate growth of neurofibromas?A survey on 59 NF1 patients. *BMC Cancer*, 5, 16.
[121] Skinner, H.G., Michaud, D.S., Colditz, G.A.,Giovannucci, E.L., Stampfer, M.J.,Willett, W.C., Fuchs, C.S. (2003). Parity, reproductive factors, and the risk of pancreatic cancer in women.Cancer Epidemiol. *Biomarkers Prev*, 12(5),433-8.
[122] NavarroSilvera, S.A., Miller, A.B., Rohan, T.E. (2005).Hormonal and reproductive factors and pancreatic cancer risk: a prospective cohort study. *Pancreas*, 30(4), 369-74
[123] Kreiger, N., Lacroix, J., Sloan, M. (2001).Hormonal factors and pancreatic cancer in women. *Ann. Epidemiol*, 11(8), 563-7.
[124] Lo, A.C., Soliman, A.S., El-Ghawalby, N., Abdel-Wahab, M., Fathy, O., Khaled, H.M., Omar, S., Hamilton, S.R., Greenson, J.K., Abbruzzese, J.L. (2007).Lifestyle, occupational, and reproductive factors inrelation to pancreatic cancer risk.*Pancreas*,Aug, 35(2), 120-9.

[125] Prizment, A.E., Anderson, K.E., Hong, C.P., Folsom, A.R. (2007).Pancreatic cancer incidence in relation to female reproductive factors: Iowa Women's Health Study. *JOP*,Jan 9, 8(1), 16-27.
[126] Teras, L.R., Patel, A.V., Rodriguez, C., Thun, M.J., Calle, E.E. (2005). Parity, other reproductive factors, and risk of pancreatic cancer mortality in a large cohort of U.S. women (United States).*Cancer Causes Control*, 16(9),1035-40.
[127] Abe, M.,Yamashita, J., Ogawa, M. (2000). Medroxyprogesterone acetate inhibits human pancreatic carcinoma cell growth by inducing apoptosis in association with Bcl-2 phosphorylation. *Cancer*, 88(9),2000-9.
[128] McGrath, M., Michaud, D.S., De Vivo, I. (2006).Hormonal and reproductive factors and the risk of bladder cancer in women.*Am.J.Epidemiol*,163(3), 236-44.
[129] Cantwell, M.M., Lacey, J.V.Jr., Schairer, C., Schatzkin, A., Michaud, D.S. (2006). Reproductive factors, exogenous hormone use and bladder cancer risk in a prospective study.*Int.J.Cancer*,119,2398-401
[130] Rossing, M.A.,Voigt, L.F., Wicklund, K.G.,Williams, M., Daling, J.R. (1998).Use of exogenous hormones hormones and risk of papillary thyroid cancer (Washington, United States).*Cancer Causes Control*, 9(3), 341-9.
[131] Custer, B., Longtreth, W.T. Jr., Phillips, L.E., Koepsell, T.D.,Van Belle, G. (2006). Hormonal exposures and the risk of intracranial meningioma in women: a population-based case-control study.*BMC Cancer*, 6,152.

HAZARDOUS PRESCRIPTION

Rosa Sabatini

General Hospital Policlinico, University of Bari, Italy

Toxic effects of the hormonal contraceptives (HCs) are rare but potentially serious and require permanent termination of their use.HCs are contraindicated if there is a personal or family history of Porphyries, systemic lupus erythematosus, erythema nouex, and polyarteritis nodosa. Combined formulations favor the formation of delta-aminolevulinic acid and should be avoided in case of Porphyrie. Drugs exposure can be a frequent precipitant of the acute attack in variegate porphyria; whereas, hormonal factors were more important in acute intermittent porphyria ($p < 0.00001$). Patients with acute intermittent porphyria also, show a trend to earlier and more frequent recurrent acute attacks following the initial admission(1,2). Acute intermittent porphyria is the most common type of porphyria.Its characteristic feature is periods of remissions and aggravations. Aggravation or an attack of the disease may be caused by many endogenous and exogenous factors, among others by hormonal contraceptives. The attack included abdominal pain, vomiting, reduction in muscle strength in limbs and it was complicated by seizures caused by hyponatraemia. High excess haem precursors in urine was observed. In a described case there were a few porphyrogenous factors whose action was observed, among which the most important was desogestrel.(3,4) Due to this conclusion, a change in contraceptive therapy that would exclude hormonal contraception was suggested. Polyarteritis nodosa has been progressive illness resulting in a systemic necrotizing vasculitis which may affect the kidneys, gastrointestinal tract, skin, nerves and ,muscles (5).Systemic lupus erythematous usually affects young women of reproductive age. Pregnancy may be possible if conception occurs during a stable remission of at least 6 months. Therefore, it is mandatory to avoid the estrogens because of the high vascular risk and the possibility of an exacerbation of the disease. Low-dose progestins or progestin-releasing IUDs appear the logical choose for these women(6) .Focal nodular hyperplasia of liver is less dangerous than hepatic adenomas but still necessitate stopping use.This pathological entity had been reported in women prior to widespread use of the pill,but HCs use appear to favor its growth and the development of subhepatic vein thrombosis or the Budd-Chiari syndrome,due primarily to the pill-estrogen content,as reported in sporadic cases(7,8). Estrogen-containing contraceptive methods are contraindicated in patients with acute liver diseases(9)Cerebral vein and sinus thrombosis is a relatively uncommon condition affecting young women, that may occur in HC users affected by congenital thrombophilia,especially if prothrombotic conditions as nephrotic syndrome , hyperhomocysteinemia or if unknown dural arteriovenous malformations are presents;however, the causal relationship is not well established(10,11).Fortunately, these findings are reported only in sporadic cases. It is essential to provide the preventive diagnosis with the aim to avoid a probable

high risk for the woman.The thrombotic risk , particularly of third-generation oral contraceptives use;was reported elevated among carriers of the factor V Leiden mutation(a hereditary disorder in which activated factor V is inactivated by activated protein C- APC).This disorder is a common risk factor for venous thrombosis,which is associated with a 3-to 7-fold increased risk in heterozygous individuals. Rosing reported that oral contraceptives use lead to acquired activated protein C(APC) resistance and women using third generation HC are more resistant to the anticoagulant action of APC than users of second-generation

HCs(12,13). Particularly, a report showed the occurrence of vena cava inferior thrombosis,renal vein thrombosis and pulmonary embolism due to inherited protein C deficiency in a 18-year old woman treated with HCs for three months(14). Similarly, cases of Budd-Chiari Syndrome in carriers of antithrombin III deficiency with a current or past history of oral contraceptive use had been reported(15,16) The increase in blood pressure associated with HCs administration is generally mild and usually seen during the first or the second year of use. It is prudent to monitor blood pressure at least every 6 months in women receiving combined hormonal contraceptives, and it is mandatory in women over 35. Furthermore, it is important to consider if the woman smokes or if she has some lipid anomalies.In fact, women who take HCs have an increased risk of developing new hypertension, which returns to baseline within 1 to 3 months of HC cessation(17). However, some cases of irreversible hypertension, kidney failure and malignant nephrosclerosis have been reported(18,19). Women with pre-existing hypertension who take HCs have an increased risk of stroke and myocardial infarction when compared with hypertensive women who do not(20).Most women with congenital cardiac disease can safely use oral contraceptives,especially low-estrogen combination or progestin-only preparations.Clearly, oral contraceptives should be avoided in all patients at particular risk of thromboembolic complications because of pulmonary hypertension,Eisenmenger syndrome,rhythm disturbances,reduced ventricular function,arterial hypertension , infectious complications (endocarditis)or hyperlipidemia. Intrauterine devices are very effective, have no metabolic side effects and merely carry a small risk of endocarditis.Newer devices containing progesterone only may put the patients at a still smaller risk.Contraceptive subdermal implants (e.g. levonorgestrel) are used with good results in the United States for patients with contraindications to estrogen-containing oral contraceptives (21) Smoking increases the risk of hypertension by some 2 to 3 times.Smoking increases the risk of vascular damage by increasing sympathetic tone, platelet stickness and reactivity, free radical production, damage of endothelium ,and by surges in arterial pressure(22,23).Almost 18%of the women suffering from migraine headaches and this data explains as the gynaecologyst will often be asked by their patients to prescribe hormonal contraceptives.Several evidences showed that migraine is a contraindication to hormonal contraception in all women with aura and those aged 35 or older(24). The use of highly effective reversible contraceptives is important for women with health issue,yet sometimes those same illnesses make the contraceptives themselves less effective or less safe. Common conditions are: systemic lupus erytematosus,uncontrolled diabetes mellitus, anticonvulsivant use for epilepsy or mood disorders,HIV infection,migraine headache,and obesity(25).In addition,vitamin C in amounts of 1g/day has been found to intensify the action of contraceptives by enhancing systemic estrogen action.The tuberculostatic drug rifampicin reduces the breakdown of estrogen and progestin components for oral contraceptives.Antibiotics or sulfonamides seem reduce effectiveness of contraceptives by slowing reabsorption of estrogens due to reduced intestinal microflora(26,27) The classic antiepileptic drugs(AEDs)Phenytoin, Phenobarbital, Ethosuximide and Carbamazepine reduce contraceptive effectiveness by induction of hepatic cytochrome CYP450 enzymes ,and also increase the capacity of sex hormone binding globulin(SHBG).Both estrogen and progesterone influence seizure activity in women with epilepsy, with estrogen generally demonstrating proconvulsant and progesterone anticonvulsant effects. While,hepatic enzyme inducers alter steroid metabolism in women receiving oral contraceptives, increase the risk for contraceptive failure, and interfere with calcium absorption and vitamin D metabolism, thus increasing the risk for osteoporosis and fractures. Which contraception for women with epilepsy? Combined oral contraceptives (COC) containing a high progestin dose, well above the dose needed to inhibit ovulation, and to take the " pill" continuously ("long cycle therapy"). But even with the continuous intake of a COC containing a higher progestin dose contraceptive safety cannot be guaranteed, thus additional contraceptive protection may be recommended.during the anticonvulsivant therapy. Progestin-only pills (POPs) are likely to be ineffective, if used in combination with anticonvulsivant therapy.Subdermal progestogen implants are not recommended in patients on AEDs,because of published high failure rates.Depot medroxyprogesterone -acetate (DMPA) injections appear to be effective,however, they may not be first choice due to reported side-effects(intermenstrual bleeding,delayed return to fertility, impaired bone health). The use of intrauterine devices is an alternative method of contraception in the majority of women, with the advantage of no relevant drug-drug interactions.The levonorgestrel intrauterine system (IUS) appears to be effective, even in women taking AEDs. Likelihood of serious side effects is low in the IUS users. Recommendation for women taking COC include possible use of noninducing AEDs as Valproic acid and some new AEDs (28,29,30). Nevertheless, hormonal contraception confers comparable or superior efficacy compared with such other contraceptives as the intrauterine device and barrier methods and remains an appropriate option in women with epilepsy.(31)

Ethinylestradiol –containing formulations have been shown to unmasque LSE or trigger a crisis,and can induce unwilling metabolic and/or vascular effects(6,25).Initial manifestations or exacerbations of SLE are noted during the first six months after starting HCs.However, seems that the incidence of disease flare-ups is the same ,as in patients not using HCs. However, the risk of side-effects of these preparations depend on the estrogen dose and the progestin type(32,33).In the meantime,it is mandatory to avoid combined hormonal contraception in SLE patients with high levels of antiphospholipid antibodies and, in those with active nephritis.In fact,an observational study performed on SLE-affected women, using combined oral contraceptives (COCs) reported that 22% of those suffered from thromboses during use (St.Thomas'Hospital-London) (34,35) Progestagen- only contraceptives can lead to side-effects but do not seem to activate the disease(36).Considering that expression of progesterone receptors was found in 75% of neurofibromas,it was believed that hormonal contraceptive might promote their tumor growth.This problem is very important in women affected from neurofibromatosis type1(NF 1).While ,oral contraceptives do not seem to stimulate it. However,prescription of high doses of synthetic progesterone can have this negative effect and deserve more caution(37).The combined hormonal contraceptives are absolutely contraindicated in women with acute liver and serious renal diseases(38,39,40). However, also women with familial defect of biliary excretion , including the Dubin-Johnson syndrome, Rotor's syndrome,and benign intrahepatic recurrent cholestasis should not take oral contraceptives(41). Comprehensive contraceptive counselling for HIV-1 infected women requires an understanding of the effects of various contraceptive methods on HIV-1 disease progression(42).A recent study carried out on 4549 women.aged 15-24 in four African countries reports that users of DMPA have a significantly, higher seroprevalence than non users;while,oral contraceptives and traditional methods did not show any risk for HIV(43).On the contrary,other investigators affirmed that DMPA did not affect CD4+ counts or HIV RNA levels(44).Besides,another study performed in Zambia on 599 post-partum women,HIV-infected shows that clinical disease progression(death or CD4+ lymphocyte count dropping below 200 cells/ microL) was more common in hormonal contraceptive users(13.2/100 woman-years)than in IUD users(45).This observation requires caution and urgent further studies.In addition,it is important to remember that antiretroviral regimens containing protease inhibitors and non-nucleoside reverse transcriptase inhibitors may decrease the levels of steroids released by hormonal contraceptives(46).

REFERENCES

[1] Hift, R.J., Meissner, P.N. (2005). An analysis of 112 acute porphyric attacks in Cape Town, South Africa: Evidence that acute intermittent porphyria and

variegate porphyria differ in susceptibility and severity. *Medicine (Baltimore)*.Jan, 84(1), 48-60

[2] Bianketti, J., Lipniacka, A., Szlendak, U., Gregor, A. (2006). [Acute intermittent porphyria and oral contraception. *Case report] Ginekol Pol*, Mar,77(3), 223-6

[3] Andersson, C., Innala, E., Backstrom, T. (2003). Acute intermittent porphyria in women: clinical expression, use and experience of exogenous sex hormones. A population-based study in northern Sweden.*J Intern Med*, 254(2), 176-83. *Horm.Metab.Res*, 199527(8), 379-83.

[4] Gross, U., Honcamp, M., Daume, E., Frank, M., Dusterberg, B., Doss, M.O. (1995). Hormonal oral contraceptives, urinary porphyrin excretion and porphyrias. *Horm.Metab.Res,*27(8), 379-83.

[5])Pettigrew, H.D.,Teuber, S.S., Gershwin, H.B. (2007). Polyarteritis nodosa.Compr. *Therapy*, 33(3), 144-9.

[6] Musson, P., Serfaty, D., Puissant, A. (1985). Contraception in women suffering from systemic lupus erythematous. *Contracept.Fertil. Sex (Paris),*13(10), 1063-7.

[7] Shilling, M.K., Zimmermann, A., Radaelli, C., Seiler, C.A., Buchler, M.W. (2000). Liver nodules resembling focal nodular hyperplasia after hepatic venous thrombosis.*J.Hepatol*,33(4), 673-6.

[8] Shortell, C.K., Schwartz, S.I. (1991). Hepatic adenoma and focal nodular hyperplasia.*Surg. Gynecol.Obstet*, 173(5), 426-31.

[9] Connolly, T.J., Zuckerman, A.L. (1998). Contraception in the patient with liver disease. *Semin.Perinatol*, 22(2), 178-82

[10] De Freitas, G.R. (2008). Bogousslavsky J.Risk factors of cerebral vein and sinus thrombosis. *Front. Neurol.Neurosci*, 23,23-54.

[11] Khatri, I.A., Al Kawi, A., Ilyas, A., Ilyas, M.S. (2006). Unusual causes of cerebral venous thrombosis. *J.Pak.Med.Assoc*, 56(11), 501-6.

[12] Aparicio, C., Dahlback, B. (1996).Molecular mechanisms of activated protein C resistance: properties of factor V isolated from an individual with homozygosity for the Arg506 to Gln mutation in the factor V gene.*Biochem.J,* 313, 467-472.

[13] Rosing, J., Tans, G., Nicolaes, G.A.et al. (1997).Oral contraceptives and venous thrombosis: different sensitivities to activated protein C in women using second-and third-generation oral contraceptives.*Br.J Haematol*, 97, 233-238

[14] Gundersen, T., Gjennestad, A.L., Odegaard, O.R. (1991). Protein C deficiency and the pill. *Tidsskr Nor Laegrforen*, 111(10), 1245-6.

[15] McClure, S., Dinscsoy, H.P., Glueck, H. (1982). Budd-Chiari Syndrome and antithrombin III deficiency. *Am.J.Clin.Pathol*, 78(2), 236-41.
[16] Akbas, T., Imeryuz, N., Bayalan, F., Baltacroglu, F., Atagunduz, P., Mulazimoglu, L., Direskenell, H. (2007). A case of Budd-Chiari syndrome with Behcet's disease and oral contraceptive usage. *Rheumatol.Int*, 28(1), 83-86.
[17])Atthobari, J., Gansevoort, R.T., Visser, S.T., De Jong, P.E., De Jong –van den Berg, L.T. (2007). Prevend Study Group. The impact of hormonal contraceptives on blood pressure, urinary albumin excretion and glomerular filtration rate. *Br. J. Clin. Pharmacol*, 63(2), 224-31.
[18] Lin, K.G., Isies, C.G., Hodsman, G.P., Lever, A.F., Robertson, J.W. (1987). Malignant hypertension in women of childbearing age and its relation to the contraceptive pill. *Br. Med. J. (Clin. Res. Ed.)*, 294(6579), 1057-9.
[19] Riera, M., Navas–Parejo, A., Gomez, M., Cerezo, S. (2004). Malignant hypertension and irreversible kidney failure associated with oral contraception pill intake. *Nefrologia*, 24(3), 298-9.
[20] Kelleher, C.C. (1991). Cardiovascular risks of oral contraceptives: dose-response relationship. *Contracept. Fertil. Sex*, 19(4), 285-8.
[21] Seifert-Klauss, V., Kaemmerer, H., Brunner, B., Schneider, K.T., Hess, J. (2000).Contraception in patients with congenital heart defects. *Z.Kardiol*, 89(7), 606-11.
[22] Shen, Q., Lin, D., Jiang, X., Li, H., Zhang, Z. (1994). Blood pressure changes and hormonal contraceptives. *Contraception*, 50(2), 131-141.
[23] Pollara, T., Kelsberg, G., Safranek, S., Schrager, S. (2006). Clinical inquiries. What is the risk of dverse outcomes in a woman who develops mild hypertension from OC s? *J. Fam. Pract*, 55(11), 986-8.
[24] Loder, C., Rizzoli, P.,Goiuo, J. (2007). Hormonal management of migraine associated with menses and the menopause:a clinical review *Headache*, 47(2), 329-40.
[25] Teaf, S.S., Ginosar, D.M. (2007).Contraception for women with chronic medical conditions. *Obstet. Gynecol.Clin.North Am*, 34(1), 113-26.
[26] Fotherby, K. (1990). Interactions with oral contraceptives. *Am.J.Obstet.Gynecol*, 163(6), 2153-9.
[27] Werner-Zodrow, I. (1986). Interactions of drugs with oral contraceptives.*Gynakol.Rundsch*, 26(Suppl.1), 7-17.
[28] Schwenkhagen, A.M., Stodieck, S.R. (2008). Which contraception for women with epilepsy? *Seizure*, 17(2), 145-50.
[29] Montouris, G. (2007). Importance of monotherapy in women across the reproductive cycle. *Neurology*, 69(24 Suppl 3), S10-6.

[30] Bozhinova, S., Bozhinov, P., Porozhanova, V. (2001). Hormonal contraception and epilepsy. *Akush Gynekol (Sofia)*, 42(2), 18-21.
[31] Zupanc, M.L. (2006).Antiepileptic drugs and hormonal contraceptives in adolescent women with epilepsy. *Neurology*, 66(6 Suppl 3), S37-45.
[32] Jungers, P., Liote, F., Dehaine, V., Dougados, M.,Viriot, J., Pelissier, C., Kuttenn, F. (1990). Hormonal contraception and lupus. *Ann.Med. Interne(Paris)*, 141(3), 253-6.
[33] Sammaritano, L.R. (2007). Therapy insight :guidelines for selection of contraception in women with rheumatic diseases. *Nat.Clin.Pract.Rheumatol*, 3(5), 273-81.
[34] Jungers, P., Dougados, M., Pèlissier, C., Kuttenn, F., Tron, F., Pertuiset, N., Bach, J.F. (1982). Effect of hormonal contraception on the course of lupus nephropathy. *Nouv.Presse Med*, 11(51), 3765-8.
[35] Lakasing, L., Khamashta, M. (2001). Contraceptive practices in women with systemic lupus erythematous and/or antiphospholipid syndrome :what advice should we be giving? *J.Fam. Plann.Reprod.Health Care*, 27(1), 7-12
[36] Julkunen, H.A. (1991). Oral contraceptives in systemic lupus erythematosus: side-effects and influence on the activity of SLE. *Scand.J. Rheumatol*, 20(6), 427-33.
[37] Lammert, M., Mautner, V.F., Kluwe, L. (2005). Do hormonal contraceptives stimulate growth of neurofibromas? A survey on 59 NF1 patients.*BMC Cancer*, 5, 16.
[38] Connolly, T.J., Zuckermann, A.L. (1998).Contraception in the patient with liver disease.Semin. *Perinatol*, 22(2), 178-82.
[39] Bradley, J.R., Reynolds, J.,Williams, P.D., Appleton, D.S. (1986). Encephlopathy in renovascular
[40] hypertension associated with the use of oral contraceptives.*Postgrad. Med. J*, 62(733),1031-3.
[41] Girndt, J. (1978). Oral contraceptives, hypertension and nephrosclerosis. *Fortschr.Med*, 96(7), 327-32.
[42] Lindberg, M.C. (1992). Hepatobiliary complications of oral contraceptives. *J.Gen.Intern.Med*,7(2), 199-209.
[43] Richardson, B.A., Otieno, P.A., Mbori-Ngacha, D., Overbaugh, J., Farquhar, C., John-Stewart, G.C. (2007). Hormonal contraception and HIV-1 disease progression among post-partum Kenyan women. *AIDS*, 21(6),749-53.
[44] Leclerc, P.M., Dubois-Colas, N., Garenne, M. (2008). Hormonal contraception and HIV prevalence in four African countries.*Contraception*,77(5), 371-6.

[45] Watts, D.H., Park, J.G., Cohn, S.E.,Yu S., Hitti, J., Stek, A.,Clax P.A., Muderspach, L., Lertra, J.J. (2008). Safety and tolerability of depot medroxyprofesterone acetate among HIV-infected women on antiretroviral therapy:ACTG A5093.*Contraception,*77(2), 84-90.
[46] Stringer, E.M., Kaseba, C., Levy, J., Sinkala, M.,Goldenberg, R.L.,Chi, B.H., Matongo, I.,Vermund, S.H., Mwanahmuntu, M., Stringer, J.S. (2007). A randomized trial of the intrauterine contraceptive device vs hormonal contraception in women who are infected with the human immunodeficiency virus. *Am.J.Obstet.Gynecol*,197(2), 144-8.
[47] El-Ibiary, S.Y.,Cocohoba, J.M. (2008). Effects of HIV antiretrovirals on the pharmacokinetics of hormonal contraceptives. *Eur. J. Contracept. Reprod. Health Care*, 13(2), 123-32.

HORMONAL CONTRACEPTION IN FEMALE TRANSPLANT RECIPIENTS

In the last years, the surgical progress led to progressive increase of number and survival time of transplant female recipients. Oral and intrauterine device contraceptives are generally,considered contraindicated, but if pregnancy occurs in the first year after transplantation, the survival graft may be in danger. While, the quality of life of these women,including sexuality and childbearing, have become important issues.

Hormonal contraception in female kidney recipients

The choice of an optimal contraception free-risk, is difficult in allograft recipient woman,even when successful renal transplantation restores normal menstrual cycle and fertility, in previously uremic patients(1).In fact,ovulatory cycles are observed in 72% of these patients (2). In fact, post-transplant diabetes, osteonecrosis, cataracts, and nephrotoxicity may be directly related to the various immunosuppressive drugs currently used. The lowest dose compatible with graft acceptance should help reduce the incidence of these nonfatal but significant complications. Patients with a lower glomerular filtration rate are more susceptible to the development of secondary hypertension and worse graft survival (3).The development of the graft nephroarteriosclerosis, as a consequence of hypertension may accelerate the progression of the post-transplant nephropathy(4) Adequate counseling on contraception is imperative in order to avoid unwanted pregnancies. In fact, if pregnancy occur too soon after transplantation,the survival graft is in danger.(1) Nevertheless these contraindication to hormonal contraception, in women showing stable graft function and without other risk factors,effective hormonal contraception may be considered(5). A study carried out on twenty six women with mean serum creatinine of 1.3 mg/dl ,taking combined oral contraceptives(20-35 mcg EE and 3th generation of progestins) versus contraceptive patch(20mcg EE and 150mcg norelgestromin) reported good cycle control and high acceptability Oral contraceptives were discontinued in two cases: in one because of deep thrombophlebitis and in another case because of deterioration of liver function. No other side-effects were reported,.until the end of study(18 months) Hormonal contraception did not significantly influence body mass index ,blood pressure,serum creatinine,or other biochemical parameters.Although, in the first year post-transplant blood pressure may be a non-immunological risk factor in long term graft survival (6).Adequate counseling on contraception is imperative in order to avoid unwanted pregnancies and to delay parenthood for at least 1 year. Premature delivery is the major problem in these patients and can be avoided by maintaining adequate graft function and controlling hypertension and infections (7).

REFERENCES

[1] Rongières-Bertrand, C., Fernandez, H. (1998).Contraceptive use in female transplant recipients. *Contracept.Fertil.Sex*, 26(2), 845-50.

[2] Pietrzak, B.,Wielgos, M., Kaminski, P., Jabiry-Zieniewicz, Z., Bobrowska, K. (2006). Menstrual cycle and sex hormone profile in kidney-transplanted women.*Neuro Endocrinol.Lett*,27(1-2), 198-202.

[3] Fernandez-Fresnedo, G., Palomar, R., Escallada, R., Martin de Francisco, A.L., Cotorruelo, J.G., Zubimendi, J.A., Sanz de Castro, S., Ruiz, J.C., Rodrigo, E., Arias, M. (2001). Hypertension and long-term renal allograft survival:effect of early glomerular filtration rate. *Nephrol.Dial. Transplant*, 16(1),105-9.

[4] Fabrega, A.J., Lopez –Boado, M.,Gonzales, S. (1990). Problems in the long-term renal allograft recipient. *Crit. Care Clin*, 6(4), 979-1005.

[5] Pietrzak, B., Kaminski, P.,Wielgos, M., Bobrowska, K., Durlik, M. (2006). Combined oral contraception in women after renal transplantation.*Nuuro Endocrinol.Lett*, 27(5), 679-82.

[6] Pietrzak, B., Bobrowska, K., Jabiry-Zieniewicz, Z., Kaminski, P.,Wielgos M., Pazik, J., Durlik, M. (2007).Oral and transdermal hormonal contraception in women after kidney transplantation.*Transplant. Proc*, 39(9), 2759-62.
[7] Oko, A., Idasiak-Piechocka, I., Czekalski, S. (2001). Post-transplant nephropathy and arterial hypertension. *Przegl. Lek*, 58(9), 859-63.

Hormonal contraception in female liver transplant recipients

The incidence of menstrual irregularities is high before transplantation because of chronic liver disease. While,after graft transplant ,a restoration of normal menstrual pattern is observed and pregnancy can occur(1). About 70% of transplanted women were sexually active after transplantation and 70% of those refer satisfaction with their relationship(2)It is suggested that contraception might be used at least six months after transplantation.Hormonal contraceptives may be administered as soon as liver transplant function is stable. Furthermore,some data suggest that in long-term liver transplant survivors,the risk of deteriorating liver function and eventual failure after five years remains only in those experiencing a viral hepatitis infection(3,4). A recent,preliminary study suggested that low-dose combined hormonal contraceptives(COCs) are well tolerated and did not seem to impair graft function (5).However,considering the vital importance of draft organ in these women,it is advisable that further multicenter studies are performed in this field. In fact,it is mandatory to estimate the rate of increased risk related to COC, in a larger number of graft recipients, before of a systematical use of these preparations, in the first year after liver transplantation and following.

REFERENCES

[1] De Koning, N.D., Haagsma, E.B. (1990).Normalization of menstrual pattern after liver transplantation: consequences for contraception. *Digestion*, 46(4), 239-41.
[2] Parolin, M.B., Rabinovich, I., Urbanetz, A., Scheidemantel, C., Cat, M.L., Coelho, J.C. (2004). Sexual and reproductive function in female liver transplant recipients. *Arq.Gastroenterol*, 41(1), 10-7.(1)
[3] Caccamo, L., Colledan, M., Rossi, G., Gridelli, B., Maggi, U.,Vannelli, A., Damiliano, I., Lucianetti, A., Paone, G., Gatti, S., Reggiani, P., Fassati, L.R.

(1998). Post-hepatitis primary disease does not influence 6-year survival after liver transplantation beyond 1 year. *Transpl. Int*, 11(1), S212-20.
[4] Von Schonfeld, J., Erhard, J., Beste, M., Mahl, M., Zotz, R.B., Lange, R., Breuer, N.,Goebell, H., Eigler, F.W. (1997).Conventional and quantitative liver function tests after hepatic transplantation :a prospective long-term follow-up.*Transpl. Int*, 10(3), 212-6.
[5] Jabiry –Zieniewicz, Z., Bobrowska, K., Kaminski, P., Wielgos, M., Zieniewicz, K., Krawczyk, M. (2007).Low-dose hormonal contraception after liver transplantation.*Transplant.Proc*, 39(5),1530-2.

HORMONAL CONTRACEPTION IN FEMALE HEART TRANSPLANT RECIPIENTS

In the last years, the surgical progress led to progressive increase of number and survival time of heart transplant female recipients. While, the quality of their reproductive life, assumed important relief.Counseling for contraception when sterilization is not desired, must take into account the increased risk of infection and genital carcinoma associated with immunosuppressant drug therapy (1). Teratogenicity has not been reported either with traditional immunosuppressive agents (prednisone, azathioprine) or with cyclosporine. Osteoporosis prophylaxis is particularly important in the female heart transplant recipient, because the chronic use of prednisone increases this risk. Guidelines are provided to counsel patients in these areas. (2). Generally,reproductive function improves after transplant and many cases of pregnancy had been reported in this time.The female transplant recipient attempting successful conception, pregnancy, and delivery (3,4). When the couple has completed the familial nucleus or does not desire offspring ,is important to realize whether safer method of contraception is advisable in such women. The new low-dose hormonal contraceptives can provide suitable birth control in these women but accurate and correct information about both,risks and advantages is mandatory(5).It is obligatory that the choice of a contraceptive takes into account the possible development of arterial hypertension often associated to immunosuppressive therapy and,the possible effects of the conbined formulation on coagulation and, carbohydrate and lipid metabolisms (5,6).However,a study carried-our on twenty-four female transplant recipient,before of pregnancy ,reported no side-effects during combined oral contraceptive use without the need for increasing the doses of antihypertensive drugs(6) Generally, low-dose gestagen preparations are indicated for high risk patients,while low-dosage combined preparations may be indicated for low-risk cardiac patients(7) .Therefore,choice of progestagen would be guided considering its metabolic effects.Unfortunately,hormonal contraception in heart transplant female recipients, is hitherto unresolved issue; however its use can avoid in first instance a tubal ligature.

REFERENCES

[1] Meier, P.R., Makowski, E.L. (1984). Pregnancy in the patient with a renal transplant.*Clin. Obstet. Gynecol,* Dec, 27(4), 902-13.
[2] Kossoy, L.R., Herbert, C.M.,Wentz, A.C. (1988). Management of heart transplant recipients: guidelines for the obstetrician-gynecologist. *Am. J. Obstet. Gynecol*, 159(2), 490-9.
[3] Akin, S.J. (1992). Pregnancy after heart transplantation. *Prog. Cardiovasc.Drug*, 7(3), 2-5.
[4] Maurer, G., Abriola, D. (1994). Pregnancy following renal transplant. *J. Perinat .Neonatal. Nurs*,8(1), 28-36.
[5] Spina, V., Aleandri, V., Salvi, M. (1998). Contraception after heart transplantation. *Minerva Ginecologica*, 50(12), 539-43.
[6] Seifert-Klauss, V., Kaemmerer, H., Brunner, B., Schneider, K.T., Hess, J. (2000).Contraception in patients with congenital heart defects. *Z. Kardiol*, 89(7), 606-11.
[7] Taurelle, R. (1979). Micro-pill use by cardiac patients. *Contracept. Fertil Sex. (Paris),* 7(11),789-93.

CONTRACEPTION IN WOMEN HIV INFECTED

HIV-positive women have reproductive patterns similar to those of HIV-negative women and would benefit from counselling about reversible methods of contraception. AIDS/WHO estimates that 42 million people are living with HIV/AIDS worldwide and 50% of all adults with HIV infection are women,predominantly infected via heterosexual transmission(1).Particularly, HIV/AIDS disproportionately affects young women of color(2).Recent , Highly Active Antiretroviral Therapy (HAART), with or without protease inhibitor (PI), has greatly improved the outlook for HIV-infected women,even those with an AIDS diagnosis(3) .Consequently,the dramatic reduction in HIV-related morbidity and mortality had led to a growing number of HIV-infected individuals and their partners requiring education and counseling regarding HIV-disease and reproduction(4). Assessment of options for birth control, and pre-conception counseling should be integral components of gynecologic health care for these women(5).The use of hormonal contraception by HIV-1-infected women seems to be associated with an increased risk of cervicitis and cervical chlamydia infection. HIV-1-seropositive women using hormonal contraception should be counseled about the importance of consistent condom use to prevent both sexually transmitted diseases(STI) and HIV-1 transmission (6). HIV infected womens need to be prepared to integrate contraception and gynecological care.In fact,underuse of highly effective contraception and barrier methods leaves women with HIV-infection at risk for unintended pregnancy and disease transmission(3).Was reported that among HIV-seropositive women,barrier use is more likely among women who had been pregnant(OR 1.37)and among those with higher CD4 lymphocyte counts (OR 1.10, $p = 0.0006$), whereas hormone use was linked to higher CD4 counts (OR 1.12, $p = 0.01$)(6).It is evident that in areas at high prevalence for HIV-infection,selection of longer-acting injectable contraception could be associated with lower rates of pregnancy among HIV-positive women.(7).It seems that women using the injectable contraceptive depot medroxyprogesterone acetate might be at increased risk of Chlamydia trachomatis infection (hazard ratio (HR) 3.1, $P = 0.05$) and cervicitis (HR 1.6, $P = 0.03$) compared with women using no contraception.While, the use of oral contraceptive pills could be associated with an increased risk of cervicitis (HR 2.3, $P = 0.001$). Hormonal contraception seems not associated with an increased risk of infection with Neisseria gonorrhoeae(3).HIV-1-seropositive women using hormonal contraception should be counseled about the importance of consistent condom use to prevent both STI and HIV-1 transmission. In multivariate analysis, use of hormonal ,either estrogen/progesterone oral combination or medroxyprogesterone acetate intramuscular contraceptives, high cervical mucous concentrations of interleukin (IL)-12, a positive HPV test, and persistent low-grade squamous intraepithelial lesion (LSIL) were significantly associated with the development of HSIL. The role of hormonal contraception as a risk factor deserves further investigation.(Infectious Diseases Society of America)(8).However, in the past was believed a trend between use of high –dose oral contraceptive pills and HIV-acquisition(HR 2.6), today no association was found between hormonal contraceptive use and HIV acquisition,overall.Furthermore, users who are HIV-seronegative but Herpes-simplex-virus type 2(HSV- 2)seropositive seem to have an higherrisk(9,10,11). How to promote dual protection (combined hormonal contraceptive plus condom)and how to make them acceptable in long-term relationship remains a challenge.Therefore, support for the birth control in women living with HIV is a priority(12) .

REFERENCES

[1] Mitchell, H.S., Stephens, E. (2004).Contraception choice for HIV positive women.*Sex.Transm. Infect*, 80(3), 167-73.

[2] Rove, C.,Perlmutter Silverman, P., Krauss, B. (2007). A brief,low-cost,theory-based intervention to promote dual method use by black and Latina female adolescents:a randomized clinical trial. *Health Educ.Behav*, 34(4), 608-21.

[3] Massad, L.S., Evans, C.T.,Wilson, T.E., Golub, E.T., Sanchez-Keeland, L., Minkoff, H.,Weber, K.,Watts, D.H. (2007). Contraceptive use among U.S. women with HIV. *J.Women Health(Larchmt)*, Jun,16(5), 657-66.

[4] Barreiro, P., Duerr, A., Beckerman, K., Soriano, V. (2006). Reproductive options for HIV-serodiscordant couple.*AIDS Rev*,8(3),158-70.

[5] Aaron, E., Levine, A.B. (2005).Gynecologic care and family planning for HIV-infected women. *AIDS Read*, 15(8), 420-3,426-8.

[6] Lavreys, L.,Chohan, V., Overbaugh, J., Hassan, W., McClelland, R.S., Kreiss, J., Mandaliya, K., Ndinya-Achola, J., Baeten, J.M. (2004).Hormonal contraception and risk of cervical infections among HIV-1-seropositive Kenyan women. *AIDS*, Nov 5, 18(16), 2179-84.

[7] Mark, K.E., Meinzen–Derr, J., Stephenson, R., Haworth, A., Ahmed, Y., Duncan, D.,Westfall, A., Allen, S. (2007).Contraception among HIV concordant and discordant couples in Zambia:a randomized controlled trial. *J.Womens Health(Larchmt)*, 16(8),1200-10.

[8] Moscicki AB,Ellenberg JH,Crowley-Nowick P,Darragh TM,Zu J,Fahrat S. (2004). Risk of high-grade squamous intraepithelial lesion in HIV-infected adolescents. *J.Infect.Dis*, 190(8),1413-21.

[9] Martin, H.L. Jr., Nyange, P.M., Richardson, B.A., Lavreys, L., Mandaliya, K., Jackson, D.J., Ndinya-Achola, J.O., Kreiss, J. (1998). Hormonal contraception,sexually transmitted diseases,and risk of heterosexual transmission of human immunodeficiency virus type 1. *J.Infect.Dis*, 178(4), 1053-9.

[10] Morrison, C.S., Richardson, B.A., Mmiro, F., Chipato, T., Celentano, D.D., Luoto, J., Mugerwa, R., Padian, N., Rugpao, S., Brown, J.M.,Cornelisse, P., Salata, R.A. (2007). Hormonal Contraception and the Risk of HIV Acquisition(HC-HIV)Study Group.Hormonal contraception and the risk of HIV acquisition. *AIDS*, 21(1), 85-95.

[11] Macqueen, K.M., Johnson, L., Alleman, P., Akumatey, B., Lawoyin, T., Nyiama, T. (2007). Pregnancy prevention practices among women with

multiple partners in an HIV prevention trial. *J.Acquir.Immune Defic. Syndr*, 46(1), 32-8.

[12] Delvaux, T., Noslinger, C. (2007). Reproductive choice for women and men living with HIV: contraception, abortion and fertility.*Reprod.Health Matters*, 15(29 Suppl.), 46-66.

In: Adverse Effects of Hormonal Contraceptives ISBN: 978-1-60692-819-6
Editor: R. Sabatini © 2009 Nova Science Publishers, Inc.

PART IV, MODERATE ADVERSE EFFECTS

Rosa Sabatini
Dept.Obstetrics and Gynecology,
General Hospital Policlinico-University of Bari, Italy

MODERATE ADVERSE EFFECTS HEPATOBILIARY COMPLICATIONS

Severe hepatobiliary complications secondary to the use of hormonal contraceptives are rares. Vascular symptomatology attribuitable to pill use includes the Budd-Chiari syndrome and Hepatic Peliose,which may be reversed in some cases on discontinuation of pill use (1,2,3,4).Combined hormonal contraceptives (HCs) are inducers of certain hepatic enzyme systems and their use may alter the parameters of substances such as alpha 1-antitrypsine or gamma glutamy l transferase ,with little clinical effect. HCs favor the formation of delta-aminolevulinic acid and should be avoided in case of Porphyrie(5).Reversible intra-hepatic cholestasis as estrogend ependent effect, in women with genetic predisposition may induce pruritus,anorexia, asthenia, vomiting and weight loss without fever,rash or abdominal pain. Termination of HCs clears the condition without sequelae within 1-3 months ,sometimes after a temporary aggravation. In this condition,abdominal pain and fever are most common(6).This condition is not related to duration of use and disappears 5-15 days after HC use is terminated. Moreover,estrogen-containing contraceptive methods may induce the impairement or the relief of cholestasis in liver disease such as primitive biliary cirrosis (5)Despite causing a reduction of biliary excretion,HCs may provoke jaundice which is rare and apparently due to the estrogen and the progestagen,both.Jaundice-HCs related,usually appears within the first six months of pill use and disappears ,without sequelae 1 or 2 months after termination of pill use. Half of these women developing jaundice with HCs had experienced intrahepatic cholestasis of pregnancy. These women should be closely monitored while taking birth-control pill (7). Women with familial defect of biliary excretion,including Dubin-Johnson syndrome,Rotor's syndrome,and benign intrahepatic recurrent cholestasis should not take oral contraceptives(7).Asymptomatic biliary lithiases is another possible clinical effect and is twice as common in pill users as in the control population.Therefore women taking HCs, almost always have elevated cholesterol levels in their bile which probably explains the increased frequency of complications leading to cholecystectomy,in women receiving longterm estrogen treatment. It is important to know that the anomalies in the composition of bile,almost always disappear when HCs use is stopped(8). Cholestasis induced by estrogens seems to be dose-dependet but few clinical data are available on this point.An asymptomatic lithiasis in a young HC user does not necessarily require termination of HCs(7,8,9). The role of estrogens in the genesis of hepatic adenomas is well established,but is more controversial with focal nodular hyperplasia(10,11).

REFERENCES

[1] Hung, N.R.,Chantrain, L., Dechambre, S. (2004). Peliosis hepatis revealed by biliary colic in a patient with oral contraceptive use. *Acta Chir.Belg*,104(6), 727-9.

[2] Eugene, M.,Chong, M.F.,Genin, R., Amat, D. (1985). Peliosis hepatis and oral contraceptives:a case report.*Mediterr.Med*, 13(343),21-24.

[3] Akbas, T., Imeryuz, N., Bayalan, F., Baltacroglu, F., Atagunduz, P., Mulazimoglu, L., Direskenell H. (2007).A case of Budd-Chiari syndrome with Behcet's disease and oral contraceptive usage. *Rheumatol.Int*, 28(1), 83-86.

[4] Tong, H.K., Fai, G.L., Ann, L.T., Hock, O.B. (1981).Budd-Chiari syndrome and hepatic adenomas associated with oral contraceptives.A case report. *Singapore Med, J*, 22(3), 168-72.

[5] Bianchetti, J., Lipniaxka, A., Szlendak, U., Gregor, A. (2006). Acute intermittent porphyria and oral contraception. *Case report.Ginekol.Pol*, Mar,77(3), 223-6

[6] Hecht, Y. (1991). Hepatic and biliary repercussions of estrogens:dose or duration of treatment effect.*Contracept.Fertil.Sex(Paris)*,19(5), 403-8.6)

[7] Lindberg, M.C. (1992). Hepatobiliary complications of oral contraceptives. *J.Gen.Intern.Med*, 7(2),199-209.
[8] Saint-Marc Girardin, M.F. (1984).Hepatic complications of oral contraceptives Contracept. *Fertil. Sex (Paris)*, 12(1),13-6.
[9] Leclere, J., Meot-Rossinot, B., Rauber, G. (1983).The pill and the liver. *Lyon Mediterr.Med.Med. Sud Est*, 19(2),7075-80).
[10] Shortell,C.K., Schwartz, S.I. (1991). Hepatic adenoma and focal nodular hyperplasia. *Surg. Gynecol.Obstet*, 173(5), 426-31.
[11] Tajada M,Nerin J,Ruiz MM,Sanchez-Dehesa M.,Fabre E. (2001). Liver adenoma and focal nodular hyperplasia associated with oral contraceptives.*Eur.J.Contracept.Reprod.Health Care*, 6(4), 227-30.

ADVERSE EFFECTS ON CARBOHYDRATE AND LIPID METABOLISM

Rosa Sabatini and Loverro Giuseppe

It is widely known that hormonal contraceptives(HCs) use can lead to an impairment of carbohydrate and lipid metabolism which are important risk factors for cardiovascular diseases.These effects occur with progestin-only contraceptives as well as with contraceptives containing estrogens. HCs may interfere with glucose metabolism, in part by creating an effect of peripheral insulin resistance and in part by diminishing the insulin-secreting capacities of the islets of Langerhans. It is shown that deterioration of glucose tolerance in the 1st trimester of oral contraceptives use is due to the synthetic estrogen, while hyperinsulinism after 6th month of use is due to the progestin component. The early deterioration of glucose tolerance could be due to a direct action of estrogen on the pancreas, where specific estrogen receptors have been identified. The reduction of glucose levels by estrogen is due to reduction of glucogenolysis with an increase of hepatic gluconeogenesis. These effects may be explained by the action of estrogens on insulin and glucagon: estrogen inhibit the secretion of glucagon On the other hand, progestins augment insulin and glucagon secretion without modifying their ratio in the portal vein(1,2).Hyperinsulinism is observed in women using combined hormonal contraceptives(COC) or progestins only , whether or not there is a deterioration of glucose tolerance. This effect which can appear after 3 months of use, continues as long as HCs are used. The determinations of insulin secretion are more reliable if peptide C in plasma is determined, as it is released by the pancreas in an equimolar amount with insulin and is not retained by the liver. The hyperinsulinism is due to a hypersecretion and not to a diminution in degradation of insulin. So, probable pill-induced insulin resistance is comparable to that of pregnancy(1,2,3). Although all progestins used in contraception , potentially, induce insulin resistance with hyperinsulinism,the effect seems to be largely dependent on the type of progestin used and are more marked with 19 nortestosterone derivatives than with 17 alpha hydroxy proge sterone, because of the structural similarity of 19 norsteroids (4).The most notable changes seem are seen with Levonorgestrel (LNG), mono or triphasic, and are minimal with the low-dose COC containing third-generation progestins (desogestrel and gestodene) (5,6,7). In fact, was reported that women taking triphasic combined oral contraceptives develop, after three months from the start of the treatment ,a significant increase of the plasma glucose concentration and the plasma insulin response to oral glucose.While, fasting plasma cholesterol ,HDL-cholesterol and LDL- cholesterol concentrations did not change as compared with baseline values, nor did the ratio of total cholesterol to HDL-cholesterol.While plasma triglyceride levels increased significantly (3) The effects of HCs on serum lipid levels depend on the dose of estrogen and dose and type of progestin. Generally, ethinylestradiol (EE)causes an increase in triglycerides and HDL-cholesterol, while progestins tend to increase total cholesterol and decrease HDL-cholesterol. The evaluation of impact on lipid and carbohydrate profiles of two combined oral contraceptives containing 20 mcg EE/ 100 mcg LNG and 30 mcg EE/ 150 mcg LNG showed similar effects for both preparations. Although the changes in the 20 EE group were lower compared with the 30 EE group, none of the differences between the two treatments were statistically significant(8,9). So, low-dose combined HCs seem to have slight or no effect on cholesterol, HDL-cholesterol and triglycerides but there are only minimal differences with the higher doses pill .Low-dose progestin-only pill , may have deleterious effects. Insulin-dependent diabetes in adolescents is a relative contraindication. Were investigated the eventual different effects of non hormonal contraception(NHC), combination oral contraception (COC), and depo-medroxyprogesterone acetate (DMPA) on lipids, in women with recent gestational diabetes mellitus(GDM).This observational cohort study of 972 nondiabetic, normotensive, postpartum women showed that DMPA users gained significantly more weight compared with NHC and combined HC users($P < 0.0001$). Patterns of change in LDL cholesterol, and triglycerides were not significantly different among groups. HDL cholesterol change differed only between COC and NHC groups (10).The effects of combined oral contraceptives containing low-dose ethinylestradiol associated with norethisterone,levonorgestrel or gestodene compared to copper IUDs were also evaluated in 103 women with insulin dependent diabetes mellitus(IDDM) or previous gestational diabetes mellitus (GDM).None of these women developed microalbuminuria during the study.Compared to normal women,was found reduced insulin sensitivity in the women with previous GDM using the pill(10). So,COCs can be used in women with uncomplicated diabetes and in women with previous gestational diabetes, if clinical and monitoring can be ensured. Type 1 diabetes mellitus is common in Europeans.Glucometabolic control at conception and during early pregnancy is necessary to reduce the risk of early miscarriage and congenital malformations. Safe and effective contraceptive methods are essential for these women in order to have a "planned pregnancy"under optimal conditions.Many teens lacke awareness of pregnancy-related complications with diabetes and are unaware about preconception counselling(PC).The role of PC is focused to prevent complications for women with diabetes and to offer then a highly effective birth control method for preventing an unplanned pregnancy (11,12). So ,women with diabetes need safe, effective contraception. Although intrauterine devices provide available contraception, concerns remain that progestin absorbed systemically from the levonorgestrel-releasing device may impair carbohydrate metabolism. A recent randomized study examines the effect of the levonorgestrel-releasing intrauterine system on glucose metabolism in 62 women with uncomplicated insulin-dependent diabetes mellitus.The women were randomly assigned to either a levonorgestrel-releasing or a copper T 380A intrauterine device. Outcome data were available for 29 women using the levonorgestrel-releasing and 30 using the copper device. At 12 months, mean glycosylated levels were similar for both groups.The same was registered for mean fasting-serum glucose levels and daily insulin doses (35.1 units compared with 36.4 units). No important differences were noted at either 6 weeks or 6 months(13). So, levonorgestrel-releasing device had no adverse effect on glucose metabolism, even at the 6-week observation when systemic levels of levonorgestrel would have been higher than at later observations(13). Concern about a potential adverse effect of this contraceptive on glucose control is unwarranted, and its use in women with diabetes should be liberalized .Another open-label, randomized study compared the influence on the lipid profile of two oral contraceptives containing 30 mcg EE /3 mg drospirenone (DRSP) and 30 mcg EE/ 150 mcg desogestrel (DSG). A slight increase in mean total HDL cholesterol was found for both groups, after 13 treatment cycles ; whereas, HDL2 cholesterol did not change remarkably in both groups. The mean LDL cholesterol values increased by 10.6% in the DSG group and remained nearly stable in the DRSP group(+1.8%).A slight rise in mean total cholesterol was found for all cycles after the initiation of treatment.The mean increase after 1 year of treatment was approximately 8% in both treatment groups. Mean triglyceride levels increased for both treatment groups. For total phospholipids, an increase of +13.6% (DRSP) and +18.5% (DSG) over 13 cycles was measured.In conclusion, the combined oral contraceptive EE/DRSP, as well as the reference preparation,had little impact on the lipid profile(14).Similar results of drospirenone were obtained analyzing the effects on lipid metabolism of a preparation containing 30mcgEE/ 2mg chlormadinone acetate(CMA)over a period lasting 12 cycles.The effects on the lipoproteins checked were favorable,as the atherogenic index LDL/ HDL dropped from 2.2 prior to therapy to 1.7 in 12th cycle of the treatment period.There was a significant increase in cholesterol and triglycerides , while the LDL fraction remained almost constant as for EE / DRSP. The antiandrogenic activity of the formulations containing EE/DRSP and EE/CMA may be regarded as responsible for the stable LDL cholesterol levels. As a result, the atherogenic index , ratio of total HDL/LDL was increased, a pattern that is usually considered clinically beneficial with respect to cardiovascular disease risk (15,16) .The observed changes were not suggestive of a clinically relevant deterioration of carbohydrate metabolism .The effects of Norplant compared with medroxyprogesterone acetate (DMPA) and low-dose oral contraceptive pill in diabetic women were evaluated. From this study emerged that DMPA and combined formulation-pill fasting blood sugar,while total cholesterol and LDL-cholesterol decreased in all groups except DMPA where it increased. Triglyceride only increased in pill-group. HDL-cholesterol increased with the pill and decreased with Norplant and DMPA.Partial thromboplastin time was prolonged in Norplant users(17).Therfore, Norplant use results in minimal metabolic alterations ,while DMPA seems to have unfavorable outcome. The vaginal hormone-releasing system(15 mcg EE,120 mcg Etonogestrel)showed in women with type- 1 diabetes, no clinically significant effects on carbohydrate and lipid metabolism with neutral impact on the hemostasis system(18,19,20)Current evidence suggests that hormonal contraceptives have limited effect on carbohydrate metabolism and glucose tolerance in HC-users, but women with diabetic risk factors may be more sensitive to the vascular impact of these formulations than others.However,strong statements cannot be made, though, due to having few studies that compared any particular types of contraceptives.Many trials had small numbers of participants and some had large losses to follow up. Most studies had poor reporting of methods.No information was available regarding the effects among women who were overweight (21).Obese women should undergo an endocrinologic and metabolic examination, in the interest of general prevention, before receiving a prescription for combined hormonal contraceptives(22).Long-term studies do not indicate any trend toward diabetes in long-term users and long-term use of COCs does not appear to increase the risk of cardiovascular disease.Either the estrogen-induced deterioration of glucose tolerance or the progestin-induced insulin resistance can lead to poor glucose tolerance or type 2 diabetes mellitus in few predisposed individuals. Considering that all HCs potentially, may induce some deterioration of glucose in the tolerance tests and increase in insulin secretion, although these changes were within normal accepted levels , accurate contraceptive counselling is necessary. In addition, it is important to remember that glucose intolerance developed during pill use is not always reversible. In women with diabetes mellitus it is very important to take in account such factors as type of the diabetes,its lasting, degree of metabolic compensation, presence of diabetes complications, body-mass index of the patient and, presence of risk factors for cardiovascular diseases and future pregnancy planning(23).Women with diabetes need safe,effective contraception. Condom may be an acceptable method for some women but a high risk of user failure can be predicted.While,IUD or hormonal contraceptives may be the only reversible alternative(24,25). Combined hormonal contraceptives can have deleterious effects on serum lipids, although only persons predisposed to hyperlipidemia are truly at risk.Concern about a potential adverse effect on glucose control of the contraceptive use in women with uncomplicated diabetes is non realistic.So, hormonal contraception use is appropriate and convenient for women with controlled diabetes type 1 and 2 who do not smoke and who do not have other risk factors for cardiovascular diseases. In fact, acute myocardial infarction may occur in young women taking hormonal contraceptives who have poor metabolic state(26). It is advisable in these cases prescribe low-dose HC(pill or vaginal ring) or combination containing progestins with moderate antiandrogenic activity.In diabetic women who smoke,and in women with type 1 diabetes levonorgestrel – intrauterine device should be liberalized.To take in account the integration with diabetes control(medical or dietetic)and a weight control are mandatory.Particularly , primary preconception counseling for type 1 diabetes is convenient might be performed in the adolescent patients(27,28,29).

REFERENCES

[1] Hilal. (1985).Oral contraception and carbohydrate metabolism-the physiopathological explanation. *Contracept.Fertil. Sex.(Paris).* 13(12), 1213-7.

[2] Elkind-Hirsch, K., Goldzieher, J.W. (1994). *Metabolism:carbohydrate metabolism*.In : Goldzieher, J.W., Fotherby, K.editors.Pharmacology of contraceptive steroids.New York, USA:Raven Press, p.345-56.

[3] Sheu, W.H., Hsu, C.H.,Chen, Y.S., Jeng, C.Y., Fuh, M.M. (1994). Prospective evaluation of insulin resistance and lipid metabolism in women receiving oral contraceptives.*Clin. Endocrinol*,(Oxf) 40(2), 249-55.

[4] Godsland, I.F.,Crook, D., Simpson, R. (1990).The effects of different formulations of oral contraceptives agents on lipid and carbohydrate metabolism. *N.Engl.J.Med*, 323,1375-81.

[5] Rubio-Lotvin, B. (1996).Oral hormonal contraceptives and carbohydrate metabolism. *Ginecol. Obstet. Mex*, 64, 198-200.

[6] Crook, D.,Godsland, I.F.,Worhington, M., Felron, C.V., Proudler, A.J., Stevenson, J.C. (1993). A comparative metabolic study of two low-estrogen dose oral contraceptives containing desogestrel or gestodene progestins.*Am.J.Obstet.Gynecol*, 169,1183-9.

[7] Petersen, K.R., Skouby, S.O., Jepsen, P.V., Haaber, A.B. (1996). Diabetes regulation and oral contraceptives.Lipoprotein metabolism in women with insulin dependent diabetes mellitus using oral contraceptives. *Ugerskr.Laeger*, 158(17),2388-92.

[8] Endrikat, J., Klipping, C., Cronin, M., Gerlinger, C., Ruebig, A., Schmidt, W., Düsterberg, B. (2002).An open label, comparative study of the effects of a dose-reduced oral contraceptive containing 20 microg ethinyl estradiol and 100 microg levonorgestrel on hemostatic, lipids, and carbohydrate metabolism variables. *Contraception*, Mar, 65(3), 215-21.

[9] Skouby, S.O., Endrikat, J., Düsterberg, B., Schmidt, W., Gerlinger, C., Wessel, J., Goldstein, H., Jespersen, J. (2005). A 1-year randomized study to evaluate the effects of a dose reduction in oral contraceptives on lipids and carbohydrate metabolism: 20 microg ethinyl estradiol combined with 100 microg levonorgestrel. *Contraception*, Feb, 71(2), 111-7.

[10] Xiang, A.H., Kawakubo, M., Buchanan, T.A., Kjos, S.L. (2007). A longitudinal study of lipids and blood pressure in relation to method of contraception in Latino women with prior gestational diabetes mellitus. *Diabetes Care*, 30(8), 1952-8.

[11] Petersen, K.R., Skouby, S.O., Jespersen, J. (1996).Contraception guidance in women with pre-existing disturbances in carbohydrate metabolism.*Eur.J.Contracept.Reprod.HealthCare*, 1(1), 53-9.

[12] Charron-Prochownik, D., Sereika, S.M., Wang, S.L., Hannan, M.F., Fischl, A.R., Stewart, S.H., Dean-McElhinny, T. (2006).Reproductive health and

preconception counseling awareness in adolescents with diabetes: what they don't know can hurt them. *Diabetes Educ*, Mar-Apr, 32(2), 235-42.

[13] Rogovskaya, S., Rivera, R., Grimes, D.A., Chen, P.L., Pierre-Louis, B., Prilepskaya, V., Kulakov, V. (2005).Effect of a levonorgestrel intrauterine system on women with type 1 diabetes: a randomized trial. *Obstet Gynecol*, Apr, 105(4), 811-5.

[14] Gaspard, U., Endrikat, J., Desager, J.P., Buicu, C., Gerlinger, C., Heithecker, R. (2004). A randomized study on the influence of oral contraceptives containing ethinylestradiol combined with drospirenone or desogestrel on lipid and lipoprotein metabolism over a period of 13 cycles. *Contraception*, 69(4), 271-8.

[15] Cirkel, U., Belkien, L., Hanker, J.P., Schweppe, K.W., Schneider, H.P. (1986). Effects of a chlormadinone acetate-containing ovulation inhibitor on androgenization pictures and liver and lipid metabolism in young females. Geburtshilfe Frauenheilkd, Jul, 46(7), 439-43

[16] Zahradnik, H.P., Hanjalic Beck, A. (2008). Efficacy,safety and sustainability of treatment continuation and results of an oral contraceptive containing 30 mcg ethinylestradiol and 2 mg chlormadinone acetate,in long-term usage (up to 45 cycles)-an open label,prospective, noncontrolled,office-based Phase III study.*Contraception*, 77(5), 337-43. .

[17])Diab, K.M., Zaki, M.M. (2000). Contraception in diabetic women:comparative metabolic study of Norplant,depot-medroxyprogesterone acetate,low-dose oral contraceptive pill and CuT 380A. *J.Obstet.Gynecol.Res*, 26(1), 17-26.

[18] Grigoryan, O.R.,Grodnitskaya, E.E., Andreeva, E.N.,Chebotnikova, T.V., Melnichenko, G.A. (2008). Use of the NuvaRing hormone-releasing system in late reproductive-age women with type 1 diabetes mellitus .*Gynecol.Endocrinol*, 24(2), 99-104.

[19] Tuppurainem, M. (2004). The combined contraceptive vaginal ring and lipid metabolism:a comparative study.*Contraception*, 69,389-94

[20] Duijkers, I. (2004). A comparative study on the effects of a contraceptive vaginal ring and an oral contraceptive on carbohydrate metabolism and adrenal and thyroid function. *Eur. J.Contracept.Reprod.Health Care*, 9, 131-40.

[21] Lopez, L.M., Grimes, D.A., Schulz, K.F. (2007). Steroidal contraceptives: effect on carbohydrate metabolism in women without diabetes mellitus. *Cochrane Database Syst Rev,*Apr, 18,(2), CD006133.

[22] Gaspard, U. (1988).Oral contraception,glucid metabolism and monitoring criteria. *Contracept. Fertil. Sex(Paris),*16(2), 113-

[23] Nikolov, A., Dimitrov, A., Kolarov, G., Todarova, K., Mekhandzhiev, T.S. (2005). Contraception in women with diabetes mellitus.*Akush Ginekol(Sofia)*, 44(5), 47-52
[24] Skouby, S.O., Molsted-Pedersen, L., Petersen, K.R. (1991).Contraception for women with diabetes:an update.*Baillieres Clin.Obstet.Gynaecol*, 5(2), 493-503.
[25] Falsetti, D.,Charron-Prochownik, D., Serelka, S., Kitutu, J., Peterson, K., Becker, D., Jacober, S., Mansfield, J.,White, N.H. (2003).Condom use,pregnancy,and STDs in adolescent females with and without type 1 diabetes.*Diabetes Educ*, 29(1), 135-43.
[26] Rogowicz, A., Zozulinska, D., Wierusz-Wysocka, B. (2007).Myocardial infarction in a 26-year old patient with diabetes type 1. *Kardiol. Pol*, 65(11), 1363-6.
[27] Klinke, J., Toth, E. L. (2003). Preconception care for women with type 1 diabetes. *Can.Fam.Physician*, 49, 769-73.
[28] Diabetes and Pregnancy Grroup. (2005). Knowledge about preconception care in French women with type 1 diabetes.*Diabetes Metab*, 31(5), 443-7.
[29] Charron-Prochownik, D., Sereika, S.M.,Wang, S.L., Hannan, M.F., Fischi, A.R., Stewart, S.H., Dean – McElhinny, T. (2006). Reproductive health and preconception counseling awareness in adolescents with diabetes:what they don't know can hurt them.*Diabetes Educ*, 32(2), 235-42.

HEADACHE

Almost 18% of the women suffering from migraine headaches and, the last Classification of Headache Disorders of the International Headache Society clearly identifies an "exogenous hormone-induced headache"that could be triggered by intake of combined oral contraceptives(COCs).It is known that headache can be related to estrogen exposure,during pill intake and after hormone withdrawal an the pill free interval(1,2). Migraine in the pill-free interval of combined oral contraceptives is reported by many women. A pilot study suggest that the use of 50 μg estrogen patch during the pill-free interval may reduce the frequency and severity of migraine at that time(3). Therefore,continuous regimen- HCs (hormonal contraceptives) may represent a convenient strategy as preventive therapy reducing the frequency,duration,and intensity of attacks(4). The newest formulations influence the headache course to a lesser extent than previous hormonal contraceptives; although,migraine and pill intake are associated both, with an increased risk of ischaemic stroke.Whatever, migraine per se is not a contraindication for COCs use(5). Anyway, it is very important to remember that patients suffering from migraine with aura ,generally show a greater thrombotic risk than women with migraine without aura. Other risk factors as patient's age, tobacco use, hypertension, hyperlipidaemia,obesity and diabetes must be carefully considered ,when prescribing COCs in migraine patients. A thorough laboratory control of the genetics of prothrombotic factors and coagulative parameters should precede any decision of COCs prescription in migraine patients. Migraine has been considered to be benign,not life-threatening illness. In spite of this, several studies suggested it as a rare risk factor for ischaemic stroke. Six cases of migrainous stroke fully meeting the diagnostic criteria of the International Headache Society (HIS) were reported and all patients had migraine with aura(6).This association is still conflicting and seems to be restricted to particular subgroups as the women under 45 years of age,with migraine with aura, who smoke and use hormonal contraceptives.Furthermore,epidemiological studies disclosed the risk of stroke is raised in women who has been suffering from migraine in their younger time(7).A large cross-sectional population-based study carried out in 46,506 women using hormonal contraceptives showed a significant dose relationship between headache and estrogen;while, no significant association between headache and COCs containing only progestagen was found(1).

REFERENCES

[1] Aegidius, K., Zwart, J.A., Hagen, K., Schei, B., Slovner, L.J. (2006).Oral contraceptives and increased headache prevalence:the Head-HUNT Study. *Neurology*, 66(3), 349-53
[2] Silberstein, S.D. (2001). Hormone-related headache. *Med.Clin. North.Am*, 85, 1017-35)
[3] Macgregor, F.B., Hackshaw, A. (2002).Prevention of migraine in the pill-free interval of combined oral contraceptives:a double-blind,placebo-controlled pilot study using natural oestrogen supplements. *J.Fam.Plann. Reprod.Health Care*, 28(1), 27-31
[4] Silberstein, S.D. (1999). Menstrual migraine. *J.Women Health Gend.Based Med*, 8(7), 919-31
[5] Allais, G. De Lorenzo C.,Mana O.,Benedetto C. (2004). Oral contraceptives in women with migraine:balancing risks and benefits. *Neurol. Sci*,3, 211-4
[6] Frigerio, R., Santoro, P., Ferrarese, C., Agostoni, E. (2004). Migrainous cerebral infarction: case reports. *Neurol.Sci*, 3, 300-1

[7] Suzuki, M. (2006). Migraine and stroke.*Rinsho Shiniceigaku*,46(11), 899-901

DERMATOLOGICAL ADVERSE EFFECTS

The equilibrium of healthy skin and mucosa may be affected by pharmaceutical agents, as hormonal contraceptives(HC) causing different manifestations. Cutaneous adverse effects as melasma, photosensitivity, bullous eruptions and monilias are frequently reported in women taking hormonal contraceptives (1). Melasma or Chloasma, a dark brown hyperpigmentation, accounts for about 2/3 of all cutaneous side-effects of HCs and,appears frequently in women who have heavily pigmented nipples and eyes (2). It may occur in these women when not protected fron sunlight and regress more slowly than after pregnancy,sometimes can be definitive(3).Progesterone activity changes the biochemistry and pH of the skin and sebacious glands, thereby contributing to eruptions of acne vulgaris (4).However,it is known that anti-androgen progestin and estrogen combinations are more effective than standard estrogen and progestagen (without anti-androgen property) contraceptive pill,to trat the acne(5). Particularly, a recent study carried out in 170 adolescent girls reported as very convenient the monophasic formulation containing ethinylestradiol 30 µg and chlormadinone acetate 2 mg for the acne vulgaris management (6)Even though many believe that using combined oral contraceptives(COCs) cause hair loss,there is little evidence to support it. Alopecia is very rare and may even reflect a simple coincidence. Reactions of hypersensitivity or allergy to COC may include urticaria and eczema. Rarely, urticaria may be a life-threatening skin disease.The sympoms may range from pruritus to generalized skin eruptions, gastrointestinal, bronchial problems to systemic anaphylaxis and cardiovascular emergencies(7).Dermatologic vascular manifestations of COCs are dependent on estrogens and include telangiectasias, angiomas and livedo reticularis(8). Although livedo reticularis or racemosa is commonly seen in women with antiphospholipid antibody syndrome or can be a non-specific lesion of systemic lupus erythematosus(9,10).Several dermatological and systemic disorders may be aggravated by COCs as Hereditary angioedema, Herpes gestationis, Porphyries ,Systemic lupus erythematosus. Same condition for hidradenitis suppurativa, seborrhoea, and Fox-Fordyce disease(1) Acute intermittent porphyria is the most common type of porphyria. Aggravation or an attack of the disease is caused by many endogenous and exogenous factors, among others by hormonal contraceptives.There are few porphyrogenous factors whose action was observed, among which the most important was desogestrel.Due to this conclusion, a change in contraceptive therapy that would exclude hormonal contraception was suggested(11).Generally, HCs favor the formation of delta-aminolevulinic acid and should be avoided in case of Porphyrie.Drug exposure was a frequent precipitant of the acute attack in variegate porphyria,whereas hormonal factors were more important in acute intermittent porphyria ($p<0.00001$)(12).Sporadic cases of Porphyria cutanea tarda caused by long–term use of oral HCs were reported in the Literature(13).Severe seborrhoeic dermatitis was reported, in the last years as rare side-effect of a levonorgestrel intrauterine system(LNG-IUS) in a 36–year-old woman,which resolved completely after removal of the IUS and the topical treatment(14). Moreover,we remember that some reports have indicated the Sweet's syndrome-like eruptions as cutaneous side-effect of combined oral contraceptives.This disease is a rare immunologically mediated condition characterized by an atypical neutrophilic reaction to the hormonal contraceptives; consequently, on cessation of their use, there is complete resolution of the lesions.General malaise and fever, sometimes associated with palatal ulceration and/or migratory thrombophlebitis. accompanie these eruptions (papules, nodules and plaques) of 2-3 week duration(15,16). When facial eruption was associated, the first worned diagnosis may be rosacea fulminans but the skin biopsy may help to clarify the nature of these cutaneous lesions(17,18,19). Furthermore, cases of erythema nodosum appeared with combined hormonal contraceptive intake,disappeared with discontinuation and relapsed with resumption of the retake had been reported. Oral contraceptives, as well as many other drugs, have been associated with erythema nodosum(20,21,22). In the oral cavity.candida colonization could be detected more frequently than in vagina and the influence of hormonal contraceptives could be pointed out (23,24).Regarding this condition, apart from direct skin attack, is much discussed the occurrence of immuno-allergic reactions of the skin, considering their usual saprophytic characteristics (25). The role of hormonal contraceptives in malignant melanoma remains controversial (26).

Autoimmune Progesterone dermatitis is an uncommon disorder.It typically occurs in females due to an autoimmune phenomenon to endogenous progesterone production, but can also be caused by exogenous intake of a synthetic progestin. There was no relationships to estrogen levels. Generally, these women refer a monthly cyclic skin eruption with pruritus , just prior to her menses. Erythema multiforme appears 48 hours after intramuscular 10mg progesterone or 10 mg medroxyprogesterone(27) .However, this entity can induce a variety of manifestations including erythema multiforme, eczema, urticaria, angioedema and progesterone- induced anaphylaxis(28). A case of progesterone-induced cyclical erythema multiforme had been reported. The patient, 33 years of age, suffered from recurrent pruritic annular and target lesions on the hands, feet, and trunk and oral laceration from 1977-83. She had taken oral contraceptives in 1972 without adverse effects. The eruptions began in the 2nd half of the menstrual cycle, worsened through the luteal phase, and were at their most florid on days 2-4 of menstrution. There was no relationship to estrogen levels; however, the postovulatory progesterone peak, as indicated by serial serum progesterone levels, corresponded to the initiation of eruptions. Erythema multiforme was induced within 48 hours by intramuscular injection of 10 mg progesterone or 10 mg medroxyprogesterone; this further evoked a rise in circulating immune complexes for 48 hours(28). There was no indication that the erythema multiforme was associated with menstrual-linked herpes simplex or the use of analgesics during menstruation. Autoimmune progesterone dermatitis is often associated with prior exposure to synthetic progesterones, as in this case(29). It has been suggested that the synthetic progesterone acts as a stimulus for antibodies which cross-react with natural progesterone. The antiestrogen tamoxifern was used successfully in this case and is a valuable alternative to treatment with oophorectomy.

The cases, published until now were almost fifty ;whereas, only nine known cases of progesterone- induced anaphylaxis are reported until 2003(26).The diagnosis may be confirmed by performing a skin and/or intramuscular allergen test, using progesterone(29). These cases were successfully treated with conjugated estrogen,antiestrogen tamoxifen, danazol,gonadotropin releasing hormone analogs or oophorectomy. Allergic contact dermatitis from contraceptive patch(estradiol and norethisterone acetate) and local and systemic contact dermatitis from estradiol had also been reported(30,31).

REFERENCES

[1] Chowdhury, D.S. (1973). Oral contraceptive and dermatology.*Calcutta Med.J*, 70(7-8), 187-8.
[2] Ippen, H. (1972).Clinical aspects of pigmentation disorders due to oral contraceptives. *Arch.Dermatol. Forsch*, 244, 500-3.
[3] Deharo, C., Berbis, P., Privat, Y. (1988). Dermatological complications caused by oral contraceptives. *Fertil.Contracept.Sex*, 16(4), 299-304.
[4] Foldes, E.G. (1988). 26(7), 356-9. Pharmaceutical effect of contraceptive pills on the skin. *Int J Clin Pharmacol Ther Toxicol*, 26(7), 356-9.

[5] Miller, J.A.,Wojnarowska, F.T., Dowd, P.M., Ashton, R.E., O'Brien, T.J.,Griffths, W.A., Jacobs, H.S. (1986). Anti-androgen treatment in women with acne:a controlled trial. *Br.J. Dermatol*, 114 (6), 705-16.
[6] Sabatini, R.,Orsini, G.,Cagiano, R., Loverro, G. (2007). Noncontraceptive benefits of two combined oral contraceptives with antiandrogenic properties among adolescents.*Contraception,*76, 342-347.
[7] Lipozencic, J., Wolf, R. (2005). Life-threatening severe allergic reactions: urticaria, angioedema, and anaphylaxis. *Clin. Dermatol*, 23(2), 193-205.
[8] Sadick, N.S., Niedt, G.W. (1990).A study of estrogen and progesterone receptors in spider telangiectasias of the lower extremities. *J.Dermatol. Surg. Oncol*, 16(7), 620-3.
[9] Saurit, V., Campana, R., Ruiz Lascano, A., Ducasse, C., Bertoli, A., Aguero, S., Alvarellos, A., Caeiro, F. (2003). Mucocutaneous lesions inpatients with systemic lupus erythematosus. *Medicina(B.Aires)*, 63(4), 283-7.
[10] Weinstein, S., Piette, W. (2008).Cutaneous manifestations of antiphospholipid antibody syndrome. *Hematol.Oncol. Clin.Notth Am*, 22(1),67-77.
[11] Bianketti, J., Lipniacka, A., Szlendak, U., Gregor, A. (2006). [Acute intermittent porphyria and oral contraception. *Case report] Ginekol Pol*, Mar,77(3), 223-6
[12] Hift, R.J., Meissner, P.N. (2005). An analysis of 112 acute porphyric attacks in Cape Town, South Africa: Evidence that acute intermittent porphyria and variegate porphyria differ in susceptibility and severity. Medicine (Baltimore), Jan, 84(1), 48-60
[13] Chowaniec, O.,Wierzbieta, J. (1980). Porphyria cutanea tarda caused by long-term use of femigen. *Przegl. Dermatol*, 67(3), 349-52.
[14] Karry, K., Mowbray, D., Adams, S., Rendal, J.R. (2006). Severe seborrhoeic. dermatitis:side-effect of the Mirena intra-uterine system. *Eur.J.Contracept. Reprod.Health Care*, 11(1), 53-41
[15] Tefany, F.J., Georgouras, K. (1991).A neutrophilic reaction of Sweet's syndrome type associated with the oral contraceptive. *Australas J. Dermatol*,32(1), 55-9.
[16] Cohen, P.R. (2007).Sweet's syndrome-a comprehensive review of an acute febrile neutrophilic dermatosis. *Orphanet J.Rare Dis*, 2, 34.
[17] Notani, K., Kobayashi, S., Kondoh, K., Shindoh, M., Ferguson, M.M., Fukuda, M. (2000). A case of Sweet's syndrome with palatal ulceration. *Oral Surg.Oral Med. Oral Pathol.Oral Radiol.Endod*, 89(4), 477-9.

[18] Femiano, F., Gombos, F., Scully, C. (2003). Sweet's syndrome:recurrent oral ulceration,pyrexia , thrombophlebitis,and cutaneous lesions. *Oral Surg.Oral Med.Oral Pathol.Oral Radiol. Endod*, 95(3), 324-7.

[19] Anavekar, N.S., Williams, R., Chong, A.H. (2007). Facial Sweet's syndrome mimicking rosacea fulminans. *Australas J.Dermatol*, 48(1), 50-3.

[20] Beaucaire, G., Mouton, Y., Brion, M., M'Belepe, R., Fourrier, A. (1980).Oral contraceptives: misunderstood etiology of erythema nodosum.*Sem.Hop*,56(33-36), 1426-8.

[21] Stumbo, W.G. (1973). Erythema nodosum secondary to the use of oral contraceptive.A case report. *J.Ky Med. Assoc*, 71(7), 433-4.

[22] Winkelman, R.K. (1978). Erythema nodosum and oral contraceptive therapy. *JAMA*, 239 (14), 1437

[23] Bernardini, U.D., Pini Prato, G. (1969).Vulvovaginitis and stamatitis caused by Candida albicans and stellatoidea during administration of oral contraceptives. *Riv. Ital.Stomatol*, 24(10), 1045-52.

[24] Klinger, G., Tiller, F.W., Klinger, G. (1982).Oral and vaginal Candida colonization under the influence of hormonal contraception. *Zahn.Mund. Kieferheilkd*, 70(2), 120-5.

[25] Bourrain, J.L., Beani, J.C., Amblard, P. (1995). Candida vasculitis. *Allerg. Immunol.(Paris)*,27(10), 375-6.

[26] Krueger, G.G., Mcquarrie, H.G., Swinyer, L.J. (1977). Desiderable and undesirable cutaneous effects of oral contraceptives.*Drug Ther*.(NY),7(9), 46-8.

[27] Snyder, J.L., Krishnaswamy, G. (2003). Autoimmune progesterone dermatitis and its manifestation as anaphylaxis :a case report and literature review. *Am. Allergy Asthma Immunol*, 90(5), 469-77

[28] Wojnarowska, F., Greaves, M.W., Peachey, R.D., Drury P.L., Besser G.M. (1985). Progesterone-induced erythema multiforme. *J R Soc Med*,May, 78(5), 407-8.

[29] Kakaria N., Zurawin, R.K. (2006). A case of autoimmune progesterone dermatitis in a adolescent female. *J.Pediatr. Adolesc. Gynecol*, 19(2), 125-9.

[30] Koch, P. (2001). Allergic contact dermatitis from estradiol and norethisterone acetate in a transdermal hormonal patch.*Contact.Dermatitis*, 44(2), 112-3.

[31] Goncalo, M., Oliveira, H.S., Monteiro, C.,Clerins, I., Figueiredo, A. (1999). Allergic and systemic contact dermatitis from estradiol.*Contact Dermatitis*, 40(1),58-9.

In: Adverse Effects of Hormonal Contraceptives
Editor: R. Sabatini

ISBN: 978-1-60692-819-6
© 2009 Nova Science Publishers, Inc.

PART V, MILD ADVERSE EFFECTS

Rosa Sabatini[1] and Raffele Cagiano[2]
[1] Department of Obstetrics and Gynecology
[2] Department of.Pharmacology
General Hospital Policlinico-University of Bari, Italy

Adverse effects represent the main factors in determining acceptability and compliance with any contraceptive method. Most frequent symptoms are: weight gain,nausea,breast tenderness and menstrual disorders(1).Mild and transitory disturbances are common in the first cycles of hormonal contraception and usually disappear after this period without any problem. Women often stop hormonal contraception because of perceived weight changes(2). This suggestion affects particularly,adolescents and young women preoccuped with body image. However,it is important to remember that breast tenderness, headache, nausea and oedema also occur in the general population and during use of placebo(3,4).Is there a real evidence of weight gain? Several studies are carried out with the aim to clarify if weight increase with hormonal contraceptives is real or only a common misperception.The combination ethinylestradiolEE) 20mcg/ levonorgestrel(LNG) 100mcg seems to have no significant impact on body weight and body composition(fat mass,fat-free mass,total body water,intracellular water, extracellular water)(5). A multicenter comparative study between norgestimate (NGM) 180/215/250 mcg/EE 25mcg versus norethindrone acetate 1mg/EE 20 mcg showed that only the 0.3% of users ,in both groups,experienced a 10% increase in weight (6).A recent randomized,prospective study evaluating the incidence of side-effects in women using EE 20 mcg/LNG 100 mcg or EE 15 mcg/ gestodene 60 mcg or vaginal ring(EE 15mcg/ etonogestrel-ENG 120mcg) reported no significant weight gain into three groups. Particularly, over 1 year of treatment ,the maximum weight gain from baseline was 2,8 kg in the first group,1,6 kg in the second group and 0,8 in the thirt group(7). Another study which compared the formulations EE 30mcg/ chlormadinone acetate 2mg and EE 30 mcg/Drospirenone 3 mg showed no significant increase in body weight in both groups of adolescents considered as demonstrated in other trials(8,9,10,11).Injectable contraceptive methods are safe,reliable and worldwide used. Depot-medroxyprogesterone acetate(DMPA) is the most commonly used injectable in the United States; but during its use irregular bleeding,breast tension,weight gain and impact on bone mineral density should be taken into account.(12).However,no differences in mean bone mineral density of distal forearm between DMPA and IUD users were showed; even though DMPA induces estrogen deficiency as demonstrated with measures performed 5 days after cessation of menstruation(13).So, the relationship between DMPA and changes in bone density remains controversial despite a substantial number of studies evaluating this potential association(14).On the other hand, weight gain and decreased bone density were frequently documented in adolescents on DMPA, particularly with longer duration of use(15).In the mean time, the higher rate of adolescent's unintended pregnancy in the industrialized countries induces to accept this potential bone risk considering the absolute priority to reduce the pregnancy risk in this age group. In women with a tendency to weight gain,under oral contraceptives because of water retention ,the use of EE 20-30 mcg/ drospirenone(DRSP) 3 mg seems the ideal method to avoid this problem(9,16) The use of a LNG-IUS(intrauterine system) during five years caused no significant weight increase and the difference in weight was of the same magnitude as that of copper IUD(intrauterine device) use.(17). In addition, a cohort study of lower and middle class Brazilian copper IUD users during ten years,explains that these women tend to gain weight during their reproductive life, because of other factors(18).So,although weight gain is perceived as a disadvantage of oral contraception,no real weight increase was reported in the majority of current investigations.It is found no decrease in the reporting of symptoms with the reduction of estrogen dose,nor with use of third-generation progestins. Little variation between monophasic and triphasic formulations was reported(1). Nevertheless, the fear of weight gain with oral contraceptives can lead to noncompliance and method discontinuation. Woman need reassurance to remove such misperceptions. In fact, lack of informative communications between gynaecologist and user and mistaken knowledge may contribute to ignorance about HC and misperceptions ,particularly in adolescents (18,19).

REFERENCES

[1] Moreau, C., Trussell, J., Gilbert, F., Bajos, N., Bouyer, J. (2007).Oral contraceptive tolerance:does the type of pill matter? *Obstet.Gynecol*,109(6), 1277-85

[2] O'Connell, K.J., Osborne, L.M.,Westhoff, C. (2005).Measured and reported weight change for women using a vaginal contraceptive ring vs. a low-dose oral contraceptive.*Contraception*, 72(5), 323-7.

[3] Redmond, G., Godwin, A.J., Olson, W.et al. (1999). Use of placebo controls in an oral contraceptive trial:methodological issues and adverse events incidence. *Contraception*, 60,81-85.

[4] Coney, P.,Washenik, K., Langley, R.G., DiGiovanna, J.J., Harrison, D.D. (2001). Weight change and adverse event incidence with a low-dose oral contraceptive:two randomized,placebo-controlled trials. *Contraception*, 63(6), 297-302.

[5] Lello, S.,Vittori, G., Paoletti, A.M., Sorge, R., Guardianelli, F., Melis, G.B. (2007). Effects on body weight and body composition of a low-dose oral estroprogestin containing ethinylestradiol 20 microg plus levonorgestrel 100 microg.*Gynecol. Endocrinol*, 23(11), 632-7.

[6] Burkman, R.T., Fisher, A.C., LaGuardia, K.D. (2007). Effects of low-dose oral contraceptives on body weight:results of a randomized study of up to 13 cycles of use. *J.Reprod.Med,*52(11),1030-4.

[7] Sabatini, R., Caggiano, R. (2006).Comparison profiles of cycle control, side effects and sexual satisfaction of three hormonal contraceptives. *Contraception*, 74(3), 220-3.

[8] Sabatini, R.,Orsini, G.,Cagiano, R., Loverro, G. (2007). Noncontraceptive benefits of two combined oral contraceptives with antiandrogenic properties among adolescents.*Contraception*,76, 342-347.

[9] Foldart, J.M. (2000). The contraceptive profile of a new oral contraceptive with antimineralocorticoid and antiandrogenic effects. *Eur.J.Contracept.Reprod.Health Care*, Suppl.3,25-33.

[10] Suthipongse, W.,Taneepanichskul, S. (2004). An open-label randomized comparative study of oral contraceptives between medications containing 3 mg drospirenone/30 microg ethinylestradiol and 150 microg levonogestrel/30 microg ethinylestradiol in Thai women. *Contraception*, 69(1), 23-6.

[11] Schramm, G., Steffens, D. (2003). A 12-month evaluation of the CMA-containing oral contraceptive Belara: efficacy,tolerability and anti-androgenic properties.*Contraception*, 67(4), 305-12.

[12] Haider, S., Darney, P.D. (2007). Injectable contraception. *Clin.Obstet.Gynecol*, 50(4), 898-906.
[13] Taneepanichskul, S., Intaraprasert, S.,Theppisai, U.,Chaturachinda, K. (1997). Bone mineral density in long-term depot medroxyprogesterone acetate acceptors.*Contraception*, 56(1), 1-3.
[14] Westhoff, C. (2002). Bone mineral density and DMPA. *J.Reprod.Med*, 47(9), 795-9.
[15] Bonny, A.E., Harkness, L.S.,Cromer, B.A. (2005). Depot medroxyprogesterone acetate:implications for weight status and bone mineral density in the adolescent female. *Adolesc. Med.Clin*, 16(3), 569-84.
[16] Borges, L.E., Andrade, R.P., Aldrighi, J.M., Guazzelli, C.,Yazlle, M.E., Isaia, C.F., Petracco, A., Peixoto, F.C., Camargos, A.F. (2006). Effects of a combination of ethinylestradiol 30 microg and drospirenone 3 mg on tolerance,cycle control,general well-being and fluid-related symptoms in women with premenstrual disorders requesting contraception. *Contraception*, 74(6), 446-50.
[17] Yela, S.A., Monteiro, I.M., Bahamondes, L.G., Del Castillo, S., Bahamondes, M.V., Fernandes, A. (2006).Weight variation in users of the levonorgestrel-releasing intrauterine system, of the copper IUD and of medroxyprogesterone acetate in Brazil. *Rev.Assoc. Med. Bras*,52(1), 32-6. 1.
[18] Hassan, D.F., Petta, C.A., Aldrighi, J.M., Bahamondes, L., Perrotti, M. (2003).Weight variation in a cohort of women using copper IUD for contraception.*Contraception*, 68(1), 27-30.
[19] Hamani, Y., Scaki –Tamir, Y., Deri-Hasid, R., Miller –Pogrund, T., Milwidsky, A., Haimov-Kochman, R. (2007). Misperception about oral contraception pills among adolescents and physicians.*Hum.Reprod*, 22(12),3078-83.

IRREGULAR BLEEDING PATTERN

Irregularity in menstrual pattern is the most common clinical side-effect of hormonal contraceptives. Therefore,an objective assessment of cycle control is critical in evaluation of a new contraceptive method for its acceptance and continuation.Bleeding patterns are more predictable in users of combined injectables.Progestin-only oral contraceptives may cause increased days of menstrual bleeding as subdermal progestin implants while combined pills may cause a decrease in days of bleeding. The use of copper IUDs is associated with increased bleeding in 18-20% of users during the initial period of three months which improves with prolonged use while levonorgestrel-releasing devices significantly, decreased bleeding (1). However, most these disorders are not clinically significant,they can lead to erratic method use or even to discontinuation(2).Early and/or late withdrawal bleeding and irregular bleeding (spotting and breakthrough bleeding) occurred more frequently in women taking COCs containing very low-dose EE(15 mcg) than in those using COCs containing 20 mcg EE(3) Although vaginal ring(EE15 µg/ etonogestrel 120 µg) users reported significant better cycle control than oral contraceptives containing 15, 20 or 30 mcg EE (4,5,6) .In Milson study, breakthrough bleeding and spotting result less frequent with the vaginal ring than with the oral contraceptive containing EE 30mcg(4.7-10.4%) and intended bleeding was significantly better for all cycles with NuvaRing (68.5-56.6%) (7,8). A preliminary study reported more high acceptability in ring than in patch users (9). Good cycle control was, generally reported in combined HC containing EE 30mcg (10, 11, 12). However, the comparison between an oral contraceptive containing 20 microg ethinylestradiol and 75 microg gestodene, with a reference preparation containing 30 microg ethinylestradiol combined with 75 microg gestodene too, demonstrated that the two regimens had no difference in cycle control,efficacy,and side-effects.The occurrence of spotting and breakthrough bleeding was low and was not different between these two preparations(13).It was reported that the long-acting progestogen –only contraceptives like levonorgestrel(LNG)- releasing subdermal implants, Norplant or intrauterine devices(LNG-IUD) as well as injectable contraceptive NET-EN 200mg given 2 or 3 monthly, produced disturbances in bleeding pattern in the majority of their users. Combined injectable contraceptives containing 50mg NET EN and 5 mg estradiol valerate caused less bleeding problems with half of the users experiencing normal pattern during one year of its use (14,15). Combined low-dose pill, both triphasic and monophasic ,produce much better cycle control and almost 90% of users have normal bleeding patterns during one year of method use.. In spite of supposed advantages of triphasic pill, randomized prospective studies on triphasic versus monophasic formulation no reported significant differences in effectiveness, bleeding patterns or discontinuation rates(16). The biphasic pill compared to triphasic pill seems to have an increase of breakthrough bleeding but the choice of progestin may be more important that the phasic regimen in determining bleeding patterns (17). Yet, considering biphasic pill versus monophasic pill,extensive evidence is available for monophasic pill.Therfore, it is advisable to prefer the monophasic formulation (18) .Progestogen-only(3-ketodesogestrel) contraceptive implant (Implanon) induce variable bleeding pattern and is characterized by relatively few bleeding events resulting acceptable to most subjects(19).When long-acting implants,injectables or hormonally impregnated intrauterine systems are prescribed,women should be informed of irregular bleeding and following amenorrhoea prior to starting the method choosed(20). A study has evaluated the effectiveness on cycle control of two formulations low-dose EE combined with drospirenone 3mg or desogestrel 150 mcg and showed that it is comparable between both groups as frequency of withdrawal bleeding without negative effects on tolerability(21). A recent prospective randomized study evaluated the cycle control of three different hormonal contraceptives: EE20µg/LNG100 µg; EE15 µg/gestodene 60 µg versus vaginal ring containing EE15 µg/ etonogestrel 120 µg.The length of the menstrual cycle was normal in all cases at screening;while,the length of menstrual flow showed a statistically significant reduction,among COC 20µg EE users in comparison with the other groups.Early and/or late withdrawal bleeding were reported at cycle 3, in 19.1% and 48.9% of the COC 20 µgEE and COC15µg users,respectively and in 15.9% of the vaginal ring users. In the same time,irregular bleeding was observed in 22.5%, 35.8% and 9.5%,respectively (4).It is evident the highest prevalence of cycle control problems with the oral contraceptive very low-dose EE than with COC low-dose.The good cycle control achieved with the vaginal ring(very low-dose EE) may be the result of the controlled release of estradiol and etonogestrel from the ring which avoids daily hormonal fluctuations(22).The weekly transdermal contraceptive patch (EE 20 µg/ norelgestromin 150µg)provides effective contraception and cycle control comparable to oral contraceptives(23,24) Body weight above 90 kilograms is associated with lower efficacy. However, the incidence of breakthrough bleeding and/or spotting seems higher with the patch , only in the first two cycles(25). Much of the woman dissatisfaction because of menstrual changes can be averted by careful counseling prior to method prescription. Open dialogue explaining the potential for bleeding irregularities is crucial in this time, in order to avoid the discontinuation that place woman at risk of unwilling pregnancy.

REFERENCES

[1] Datey, S.,Gaur, L.N.,Saxena, B.N. (1995).Vaginal bleeding patterns of women using different contraceptive methods (implants, injectables, IUDs,

oral pills). An ICMR Task Force Study.Indian Council of Medical Research.*Contraception*, 51(3), 155-65.

[2] Cheung, E., Free, C. (2005). Factors influencing young women's decision-making regarding hormonal contraceptives: a qualitative study. *Contraception*, 71,426-31.

[3] Biswas, A., Leong, W.P., Ratnam, S.S.,Viegas, O.A. (1996).Menstrual bleeding patters in Norplant-2 implant users. *Contraception*, 54(2), 91-5.

[4] Darney, P.D.,Klaisle, C.M. (1998).Contraception –associated menstrual problems: etiology and management. *Dialogues Contracept*, Spring, 5(5), 1-6.

[5] Sabatini, R., Caggiano, R. (2006).Comparison profiles of cycle control, side effects and sexual satisfaction of three hormonal contraceptives. *Contraception*, 74(3), 220-3.

[6] Winkler, U.H., Ferguson, H., Mulders, J.A.P.A. (2004).Cycle control,quality of life and acne with two low-dose oral contraceptives containing 20 μg ethinylestradiol.*Contraception*,69,469-76.

[7] Bjarnadottir, R.I.,Tuppurainem, M., Killik, S.R. (2002).Comparison of cycle control with a combined contraceptive vaginal ring and oral levonorgestrel/ethinylestradiol.*Am. J. Obstet.Gynecol*, 186, 389-95.

[8] Milson, I., Lete, I., Bjertnaes, A., Rokstad, K.,Lindh, I., Gruber, C.J., Birkhauser, M.H.,Aubeny, E., Knudsen, T., Bastianelli, C. (2006). Effects on cycle control and bodyweight of the combined contraceptive ring,NuvaRing,versus an oral contraceptive containing 30 microg ethinylestradiol and 3 mg drospirenone. *Hum.Reprod*, 21(9), 2304-11.

[9] Ahrendt, H.J., Nisand, I., Bastianelli, C., Gomez, M.A.,Gemzell-Danielsson, K., Urdi, W., Karskv, B.,Oeyen, L., Bitzer, J., Page, G., Milson, I. (2006).Efficacy,acceptability and tolerability of the combined contraceptive ring,NuvaRing,compared with an oral contraceptive containing 30microg of ethinylestradiol and 3mg of drospirenone.*Contraception*, 74(6), 451-7.

[10] Creinin, M.D., Meyn, L.A., Borgatta, L., Barnhart, K., Jensen, J., Burke, A.E., Westhoff, C., Gilliam, M., Dutton, C., Ballagh, S.A. (2008).Multicenter comparison of the contraceptive ring and patch: a randomized controlled trial.*Obstet.Gynecol*, 111(2), 267-77.

[11] Sabatini, R.,Orsini, G., Cagiano, R., Loverro, G. (2007). Noncontraceptive benefits of two combined oral contraceptives with antiandrogenic properties among adolescents. *Contraception*, 76, 342-347.

[12] Foldart, J.M. (2000).The contraceptive profile of a new oral contraceptive with antimineralocorticoid and antiandrogenic effects.*Eur.J.Contracept.Reprod.Health Care*, Suppl.3, 25-33.
[13] Suthipongse, W.,Taneepanichskul, S. (2004). n open-label randomized comparative study of oral contraceptives between medications containing 3 mg drospirenone/30 microg ethinylestradiol and 150 microg levonogestrel/30 microg ethinylestradiol in Thai women. *Contraception*, 69(1), 23-6.
[14] Taneepanichskul, S., Kriengsinyot, R., Jaisamrarn, U. (2002).A comparison of cycle control, efficacy, and side effects among healthy Thai women between two low-dose oral contraceptives containing 20 microg ethinylestradiol/75 microg gestodene (Meliane) and 30 microg ethinylestradiol/75 microg gestodene (Gynera).*Contraception*, 66(6), 407-9.
[15] Biswas, A., Leong, W.P., Ratnam, S.S.,Viegas, O.A. (1996).Menstrual bleeding patters in Norplant-2 implant users. *Contraception,* 54(2), 91-5.
[16] Haider, S., Darney, P.D. (2007). Injectable contraception. *Clin.Obstet.Gynecol*, 50(4), 898-906.
[17] Van Vliet, H.A.,Grimes, D.A., Lopez, L.M., Schulz, K.F., Helmerhorst, F.M. (2006). Triphasic versus monophasic oral contraceptives for contraception.*Cochrane Database Syst.Rev*, 3, CD003553.
[18] Van Vliet, H.A., Grimes, D.A., Helmerhorst, F.M., Schulz, K.F. (2001). Biphasic versus triphasic oral contraceptives for contraception.*Cochrane Database Syst. Rev*, (4),CD003283.
[19] Van Vliet, H.A., Grimes, D.A., Helmerhorst, F.M., Schulz, K.F. (2006). Biphasic versus monophasic oral contraceptives for contraception. *Cochrane Database Syst. Rev,* 3,CD002032.
[20] Kiriwat, O., Patanayindee, A., Koetsawang, S., Korver, T., Bennink, H.J. (1998).A 4-year pilot study on the efficacy and safety of Implanon,a single-rod hormonal contraceptive Implant,in healthy women in Thailand.*Eur.J.Contracept.Reprod.Health Care*, 3(2),85-91.
[21] French, R.,Van Vliet, H., Cowan F, Mansour D,Morris S, Hughes D, Robinson A, Proctor T, Summerbell C, Logan S, Helmerhorst F, Guillebaud J. (2004).Hormonally impregnated intrauterine systems (IUSs) versus other forms of reversible contraceptives as effective methods of preventing pregnancy. *Cochrane Database Syst. Rev*, (3),CD001776.
[22] Gruber, D.M., Huber, J.C., Melis, G.B., Stagg, C., Parke, S., Marr, J. (2006). A comparison of the cycle control,safety,and efficacy profile of a 21-day regimen of ethinylestradiol 20mcg and drospirenone 3mg with a

21.day regimen of ethinylestradiol 20mcg and desogestrel 150 mcg. *Treat.Endocrinol*, 5(2),115-21.
[23] Merki-Feld, G.S., Hund, M. (2007).Clinical experience with NuvaRing in daily practice in Switzerland: cycle control and acceptability among women of all reproductive ages.*Eur.J.Contracept. Reprod. Health Care*, 12(3), 240-7.
[24] Smallwood, G.H., Meador, M.L., Lenihan, J.P., Shangold, G.A., Fisher, A.C.,Creasy, G.W. (2001).Ortho Evra/Evra 002 Study Group. Efficacy and safety of a transdermal contraceptive system.*Obstet.Gynecol*, 98(5),799-805.
[25] Burkman, R.T. (2002). The transdermal contraceptive patch:a new approach to hormonal contraception.*Int.J.Fertil.Womens Med*, 47(2), 69-76.
[26] Audet, M.C., Moreau, M.,Koltum, W.D.,Waldbaum, A.S., Shangold, G., Fisher, A.C., Creasy, G.W. (2001).Ortho Evra/Evra 004 Study Group.*JAMA*, 285(18),2347-54.

OVARIAN CYSTS

Paradoxically, it is believed that lowering the steroid dose in modern hormonal contraceptives (HCs) has been connected with a higher incidence of large ovarian follicles and cysts formation; nevertheless, the women with functional cysts have been treated with hormonal contraceptives to obtain the resolution of these cysts(1).A previous study evaluated two groups of users randomized to receive either 20 mcg ethinylestradiol (EE)/150mcg desogestrel or 35 mcg ethinylestradiol (EE) / 250mcg norgestimate. At baseline,39% of women in the first group and 31% in the second group reported at least one follicle < 35mm.At the end of second cycle of treatment,the frequency of these follicle decreased to 14% in each group Only one subject, in the higher dose EE- group developed an ovarian cyst > 35mm in diameter(46mm) that appeared during the pill-free week ,after the first cycle ,and during the second cycle of treatment showed a progressive reduction(2). While, in other investigation no differences were found between women who had hormonal treatment and those who had not. So, prospective studies revealed that functional ovarian cysts spontaneously appear and resolve equally well within 12 weeks independent of combined hormonal contraceptive or

gestagen used(3).Particularly, in the 1993,the Fertility and Maternal Health Drugs Advisory Committee of the US Food and Drug Administration (FDA) reported that the diameter of the maximum follicular structures were around 7.5

mm in the higher dose,monophasic HC group, compared to less than 15 mm in the lower-dose,monophasic HC group and about 13.5 mm for the nonuser group. Same results for multiphasic HCs. So, the Committee concluded that neither monophasic nor multiphasic HC increase the risk of ovarian cyst development(4). However, recently a study which compared effectiveness of low-dose monophasic pills with expectant management for functional ovarian cysts reported ,after one month a remission,a rate of 63.6% in low-dose group and 52.9% in expectant group and after two months 72.7% and 67.6%,respectively.There was no statistically significant difference between the two groups. Therefore, low-dose monophasic contraceptives were no more effective than expectant management in the treatment of ovarian functional cysts(5). On the contrary, it was reported that sometimes, transitory hyperprolattinemia, excessive production of the lutheinizing hormone, deficit of progesterone production may hamper the folliculorexis and induce the development of the follicular cysts (6). Therefore, in their production the major role belongs to the hypothalamic-pituitary disregulation. In this light ,the hormonal contraceptive management may be appropriate as conservative and effective treatment of functional ovarian cysts.

REFERENCES

[1] MacKenna, A., Fabres, C., Alam, V., Morales, V. (2000). Clinical management of functional ovarian cysts :a prospective and randomized study.*Hum.Reprod*, 15(12), 2567-9.

[2] Egarter, C., Putz, M., Strohmer, H., Speiser, P.,Wenzi, R., Huber, J. (1995). Ovarian function during low-dose oral contraceptive use.*Contraception*, 51(6), 329-33.

[3] Graf, M., Krussel, J.S., Conrad, M., Bielfeld, P., Rudolf, K. (1995).Regression of functional cysts:high dosage ovulation inhibitor and gestagen therapy has no added effect. *Geburtshilfe Frauenheilkd*, 55(7), 387-92.

[4] Oral contraceptive formulation and ovarian cysts:FDA committee finds no increased risk of follicular enlargement with low-dose monophasic or triphasic preparations. (1994). *Contracept.Rep*,5(1), 6-9.

[5] Sanersak, S., Wattanakumtornkul, S., Korsakul, C. (2006).Comparison of low-dose monophasic oral contraceptive pills and expectant management in treatment of functional ovarian cysts. *J.Med. Assoc.Thai,*89(6), 741-7.

[6] Kotrikadze, K.A., Gvenetadze, A.M., Sabahtarashvilli, T.M. (2006).Clinical aspects,diagnostics and treatment of follicular ovarian cysts. *Georgian Med.News*, 135, 21-4.

DEPRESSION

Few studies focused on the depressogenic properties of the hormonal contraceptives(HC) in spite of diffuse concern about mood changes(1).Several years ago,it was affirmed that most women using combined oral contraceptives(COCs) can expect minimal change in mood(2).Furthermore, the percentage of women who reported depressive symptoms seems to decline as the number of years of HCs use increase(3) .Impairment of social functioning is a significant aspect of depression distinct from the symptoms of depression(4). Cognitive –emotional factors including the appraisal of stress,loci of control and self-integration were implicated with specific patterns of negative affect and much more so for users than for nonusers (5). A study carried by Parry in 2001 hypothesized that changing reproductive hormones,by affecting the synchrony or coherence between components of the circadian system,may alter amplitude or timing relationships and thereby contribute to the development of mood disorders in predisposed individuals(6). It is known that neuroactive steroids as the gamma-aminobutyric acid receptor agonists are important in the modulation of affect and adaptation to stress(7).A recent study reported that healthy women without underlying mood or anxiety disorder who were given a low-dose combined oral contraceptives did not experience adverse psychological symptoms despite a significant reduction in neuroactive steroids. Women have the greatest risk for developing depressive disorders compared with men.In addition several biological conditions may be involved in the predisposition of women to depression,including genetically determined vulnerability, hormonal fluctuations,and a particular sensitivity to such hormonal fluctuations in brain systems that mediate depressive states.Although considering cognitive-emotional functioning for HCs users and non users seems that the use may influence the saliency rather than the nature of cognitive-emotional pattern(5). Relational events as role-stress, sex-specific socialization and disadvantaged social status have been considered to be contributors to the increased vulnerabiliuty of women to depression. In addition,it is known that a higher proportion of housewives than women going out to full-time work show depressive symptoms.It is hypothesized that several reproductive events may be related to depression as: premenstrual dysphoric disorder, pregnancy, post-partum, menopause, miscarriage, infertility,hormone replacement therapy and hormonal contraceptive use (8,9).A recent study performed on adolescent girls treated with depot-medroxyprogesterone acetate (DPMA) over a period of 12 months, showed that those do not present depressive symptoms (10).Similar results were obtained by an australian study carried out on 9.688 young women,aged 22 to 27 years,taking combined oral contraceptives. In fact, the odds ratio of nonusers experiencing depressive symptoms is not significantly different from that of COC users (OR= 0.90-1.21)(3). Another study reports that combined oral contraceptive(COC) users have more negative mood impact than vaginal ring users as well as, irritability is more frequent in COCs containing low-doseEE than in COCs containing very low-dose EE .However, irritability decreases with duration of pill-use (11).Besides,sporadic cases of panic attacks, in women who had previously experienced depression,have been reported.However,these reports regarded the combined oral contraceptives containing high doses of ethinylestradiol(50 mcg) and appeared when these users had stopped taking the pill (12). While, a recent study has demonstrated in adolescent girls taking COCs, higher prevalence of positive mood than in MPA users (13). The problem of whether or not oral contraceptives affect the psyche function of the woman is still controversial. Furthermore, the widespread presence of the depression in the industrialized countries increases the difficulty .Although the major problems found in the clinical trials were selection bias, poor assessment of preexisting mood status and unclear definition and/or measurement of depression.

REFERENCES

[1] Kulkarni, J. (2007).Depression as a side effect of the contraceptive pill. *Expert. Opin.Drug Saf*, 6(4), 371-4).
[2] Slap, G.B. (1981).Oral contraceptives and depression:impact,prevalence and cause. *J. Adolesc. Health Care*, 2(1),53-64.
[3] Duke, J.M., Sibbbritt, D.W., Young, A.F. (2007). Is there an association between the use oforal contraception and depressive symptoms in young Australian women? *Contraception*,75(1), 27-31).
[4] Bosc, M. (2000). Assessment of social functioning in depression. *Compr.Psychiatry*,41(1), 63-9.
[5] Rubino –Watkins, M.F., Doster, J.A., Franks, S., Kelly, K.S., Sonnier, B.L.,Goven, A.J., Moorefield, R. (1999).Oral contraceptive use:implications for cognitive and emotional functioning. *J.Nerv.Ment.Dis*, 187(5), 275-80.

[6] Parry, B.L., Newton, R.P. (2001). Chronobiological basis of female-specific mood disorders. *Neuropsychopharmacology*, 25(5),102-8.
[7] Rapkin, A. J., Morgan, M., Sogliano, C., Biggio, G., Concas, A. (2006).Decreased neuroactive teroids induced by combined oral contraceptive pills are not associated with mood changes. *Fertil. Steril*, 85 (5), 1371-8.
[8] Noble, R.E. (2005).Depression in women. *Metabolism,*54(5), 49-52.
[9] Burt, V.K., Stein,K. (2002). Epidemiology of depression throughout the female female life cycle. *J.Clin .Psychiatry*,63, 9-15.
[10] Gupta, N.,O'Brien, R., Jacobsen, L.J., Davis, A.,Zuckerman, A.,Supran, S.,Kulig, J. (2001).Mood changes in adolescents using depot-medroxyprogesterone acetate for contraception:a prospective study. *J.Pediatr.Adolesc.Gynecol*,14(2), 71-6.
[11] Sabatini, R.,Cagiano, R. (2006). Comparison profiles of cycle control,side-effects and sexual satisfaction of three hormonal contraceptives.*Contraception*,74, 220-223
[12] Ushiroyama, T.,Okamoto, Y.,Toyoda, K., Sugimoto, O. (1992). A case of panic disorder induced by oral contraceptive. *Acta Obstet. Gynecol.Scand*, 71(1),78-80.
[13] Ott, M.A., Shew, M.L.,Ofner, S.,Tu, W., Fortenberry, J.D. (2008).The influence of hormonal contraception on mood and sexual interest among adolescents. *Arch.Sex.Behav*, Feb.21, Epub ahead of print.

LOW LIBIDO

The changes in desire and sexual satisfaction during hormonal contraceptive(HC) use are important elements that might relate to acceptability,compliance and method continuation.Little is known about the influence of combined hormonal contraceptive on sexual functioning. Sexual side-effects have been reported in women taking HC,although no consistent pattern of effect exists to suggest a hormonal or biological determinant(1). Sexual desire most likely represent a complex and idiosyncratic combination of biological,psychological,and social effects. Overall,Literature data show that women experience positive effects,negative effects,as well as no effects on libido during HCs use(2,3,4,5).Moreover,current pill-users seem to discontinue for low libido less frequently than did users of higher dose pills(6). In the past years an important trial reported evidence that mood and sexual desire are dissociable and suggested that HCs can have direct effects on women's sexuality. Therfore,the negative effect on sexual interest found in this study was not just a result of HC induced negative mood changes(7).Furthermore , a population survey conducted among 1466 women who used different methods of birth control(oral contraceptives,intrauterine devices, condoms,natural family planning,sterilization) indicated that combined oral contraceptives (COCs) and sterilization has less negative impact on physical and psychological functioning than the other methods used(3).This evidence is in contrast to what the general public often believes.Nevertheless, with the introduction of oral contraceptives very low-dose ethinylestradiol(EE), sexual disturbances due to vaginal dryness and low desire,is a problem which comes up often(4).A recent study evaluated the effects on vaginal dryness,sexual desire and sexual satisfaction of the hormonal contraceptives low-dose EE(20µg EE/100µg levonorgestrel(LNG)versus very low dose (15µgEE/ 60µg gestodene or vaginal ring containing 15µg EE/120µg etonogestrel). After three cycles,30.4% of the participants taking oral contraceptive containing very low-dose EE,reported vaginal dryness ; while the same problem was reported in 12.7% of the COC-low dose EE and in 2.1% of the women using the contraceptive vaginal ring. In the meantime,the highest rates of negative impact on sexual well-being were reported by COC 15µg EE users and this data may be related to falling free testosterone levels.In addition,this study reported a rate of discontinuation of 22.3% with COC low-dose EE, 30.4% with COC very low-dose and 11.7% with vaginal ring(8). Indeed,cycle control and sexual satisfaction seem to be good indicators of treatment adherence and continuation;although studies on the effects of sex-steroids on female sexual behaviour have not yelded conclusions.Many reports have been established that sexual desire,in women depends on androgen levels(2,4,6,8). But, there are reports that progestins with antiandrogenic effect in COCs do not affect sexual desire. In human population,sexual behaviour is not determined so simply by the level of sexual steroids. The difficulty arises from the complex interaction among different factors influencing female sexual function as sexual relationship type, menstrual irregularities, vaginal dryness, partner attraction and sensitivity ,culture,economic status as well as life-style .

REFERENCES

[1] Schaffir, J. (2006). Hormonal contraception and sexual desire:a critical review. *J.Sex Marital.Ther*, 32(4), 305-14.
[2] Davis, A.R.,Castano, P.M. (2004).Oral contraceptives and libido in women. *Annu.Rev.Sex.Res*,15, 297-320.

[3] Oddens, B.J. (1999).Women's satisfaction with birth control:a population survey of physical and psychological effects of oral contraceptives,intrauterine devices,condoms,natural family planning,and sterilization among 1466 women. *Contraception*, 59(5),277-86.

[4] Sanders, S.A., Graham, C.A., Bass, J.L., Bancroft, J. (2001). A prospective study of the effects of oral contraceptives on sexuality and well-being and their relationship to discontinuation. *Contraception*, 64,51-8.

[5] Caruso, S., Agnello, C., Intelisano, G., Farina, M., Di Mari, L., Cianci, A. (2004). Sexual behavior of women taking low-dose oral contraceptive containing 15μg ethinylestradiol/60 μg gestodene.*Contraception*, 69, 234-7.

[6] Bancroft, J., Sartorius, N. (1990).The effects of oral contraceptives on well-being and sexuality.*Oxf. Rev. Reprod.Biol*,12, 57-92

[7] Graham, C.A., Sherwin, B.B. (1993).The relationship between mood and sexuality in women using an oral contraceptive as a treatment for premenstrual symptoms. *Psychoneuroendocrinology*,18(4),273-81.

[8] Sabatini, R., Cagiano, R. (2006).Comparison profile of cycle control,side effects and sexual satisfaction of three hormonal contraceptives. *Contraception*,74, 220-223.

[9] Bjelica, A., Kapamadzija, A., Maticki-Sekulic, M. (2003).Sex hormones and female sexuality. *Med.Pregl*, 56(9-10),446-50.

VAGINAL INFECTIONS

Fungal vaginal infections/colonisations can be divided into a symptomatic vaginal candidiasis and an asymptomatic vaginal Candida-carriage. The latter seems to be a predisposing factor for the development of a symptomatic vaginal candidiasis. The fungal organism isolated most frequently is Candida albicans, followed by Candida glabrata, which was previously also known as Torulopsis glabrata. To a lower extend, other Candida species such as Candida tropicalis and Candida krusei can be prevalent in the vulvovaginal region. Predisposing factors for vaginal candidiasis are pregnancy, diabetes mellitus or a therapy with immunosuppressive agents. Also gestagenes showed to be a pre-disposing factor for vaginal candidiasis(1,2). Divergent results concerning the predisposition to vaginal candidiasis or colonisation due to oral contraception have so far been reported. A study was undertaken to assess whether the vaginal flora was affected by the method of contraception considering two groups of female health volunteers (n = 2 x 60) who taking different oral contraceptives. Overall, in 17%

of the subjects (20/120) yeast could be cultured out of the vaginal secretions. There was no evidence for a higher rate of Candida-colonisation in subjects taking oral contraceptives. Further, there was no evidence for a relationship between the duration of the oral contraceptives use and the rate of vaginal yeast-carriage. Also the type of oral contraceptive (combination or sequential contraceptive) had no influence on the frequency of Candida-carriage. Candida albicans was the most prevalent yeast (16/20), followed by Candida glabrata (4/20) (1).One thousand and two consecutive vaginal or cervical swabs from women attending a family planning centre were cultured. Candida albicans was isolated from 13% of women using no contraception, 16% using oral contraceptives, and from 9%, 19% and 18% of those using diaphragms, intrauterine contraceptive devices (IUD) and condoms ,respectively. These differences were not statistically significant(3).Women using the IUD had significantly more Gram-positive cocci cultured than women in any other group, while those using diaphragms had significantly more Gram-negative bacilli. The clinical impression that the use of oral contraceptives led to an increase in vaginal candidiasis, was not confirmed by this study (4). To evaluate risk factors, related to sociodemographic and clinical variables, oral contraception and sexual behavior of women with recurrent vulvovaginal candidiasis, researchers in Italy compared data on 153 patients with recurrent vulvovaginal candidiasis with data on 306 asymptomatic patients (control group A) and data on 306 patients with nonrecurrent symptomatic vulvovaginal candidiasis (control group B).

Women with recurrent Candida vaginitis were more likely than asymptomatic women to have previously used any contraceptive method (odds ratio OR= 2.08 for the pill, $p = 0.0032$; OR = 4.15 for the IUD, $p = 0.0019$; OR = 2.55 for barrier methods, $p = 0.014$). They were also more likely to have used antibiotics, in the last month before the visit (OR = 2.1; $p = 0.009$), and to have more lifetime sexual partners than asymptomatic women (OR = 3.82 for 7 partners; $p = 0.009$). Patients with recurrent vulvovaginal candidiasis were more likely than those with nonrecurrent vulvovaginal candidiasis to have used low-dose oral contraceptives (OCs) (OR = 1.59; $p = 0.036$) and to have a higher rate of monthly intercourse in the last 6 months (OR = 2.51 for 10 times; $p = 0.048$). The attributable risk of hormonal contraceptives (HCs) use for recurrent vulvovaginal candidiasis was insignificant (11-12%). However, these results can suggest that HCs may influence the recurrence of symptomatic vulvovaginal candidiasis (5).

REFERENCES

[1] Bernardini, U.D., Pini Prato, G. (1969).Vulvovaginitis and stamatitis caused by Candida albicans and stellatoidea during administration of oral contraceptives. *Riv. Ital.Stomatol*, 24(10), 1045-52.
[2] Klinger, G., Tiller, F.W., Klinger, G. (1982). Oral and vaginal Candida colonization under the influence of hormonal contraception. *Zahn.Mund. Kieferheilkd*, 70(2),120-5.
[3] Schmidt, A., Noldechen, C.F., Mendling, W., Hatzmann, W., Wolf, M.H. (1997). Oral contraceptive use and vaginal candida colonization .*Zentralbl Gynakol*, 119(11), 545-9.
[4] Peddie, B.A., Bishop, V., Bailey, R.R., McGill, H. (1984). Relationship between contraceptive method and vaginal flora. *Aust.N. Z. J. Obstet.Gynaecol*.
[5] Spinillo, A., Capuzzo, E., Nicola, S., Baltaro, F., Ferrari, A., Monaco, A. (1995). The impact of oral contraception on vulvovaginal candidiasis. *Contraception*, May, 51(5), 293-7

NEW PERSPECTIVES IMMUNOCONTRACEPTION

The world's population is a growing problem of significant magnitude affecting development. Besides, unintended pregnancies resulting in elective abortions continue to be a major public health issue. In over half of these pregnancies, women have used some type of contraception but the inconsistent use or the scarce safety of method or intrinsic causes led to conception. It has been widely hoped that immunological methods of fertility regulation by active immunization against specific antigens of the oocyte,sperm,zygote and early embryo, and the placental pregnancy hormone human chorionic gonadotropin (HCG), will provide a means to control the problem of world wide population growth. This idea of vaccine based on HCG immunogens led to several doubts because of its mechanism of action. In fact ,it interfered with the hormone-receptor, which causes reduction in the function of the corpus luteum and expulsion of the perimplantation blastocyst. The abortfacient approach on the HCG based contraceptive vaccine limited its applications in many parts of the world(1)

Researchers aim to effect an immune attack on events linked to sperm-ovum contact and fertilization. Sperm vaccine research is not as advanced as that of ovum vaccine research; although almost all studies in this field has occurred in animals with varying degrees of success. However, research in zona pellucida vaccine development must overcome the risk of immune damage to ovarian oocytes,subsequent development of autoimmune oophoritis, and disturbed ovarian function.The WHO vaccine directed against the C-terminal peptide of beta-HCG induces a specific and safe immune response. The phase 1 trial showed that this vaccine exceeded the threshold of antibody production needed to achieve protection against pregnancy(2).Contraceptive vaccine(CV) may provide viable and valuable alternatives that can fulfil most, if not all, properties of an ideal contraceptive. The development of vaccines for contraception is an exciting proposition. The molecules that are being explored for CV development either target gamete production(gonadotropin releasing hormone, follicle-stimulating hormone and luteinising hormone),gamete function (zona pellucide (ZP) proteins and sperm antigens)or gamete outcome (human chorionic gonadotropin (HCG)).Disadvantages of CVs targeting gamete production are that they affect sex steroids and/or show only a partial effect in reducing fertility. CVs targeting gamete function are better choices. Vaccines based on ZP proteins are quite efficacious in producing contraceptive effects. However,they invariably induce oophoritis affecting sex steroids.Antisperm antibody-mediated immunoinfertility provides a naturally occurring model to indicate how an antisperm vaccine will work in humans. The HCG vaccine is the first vaccine submitted to phase 1 and 2 clinical trials in humans. Sperm constitute the most promising and exciting target for CV(3). Epididymal protease inhibitor(Eppin), a gene on human chromosome 20 expressing three mRNAs encoding ,two isoform of a cystine-rich protein.Eppin 1 is expressed only in the testis and in the epididymis, Eppin 2 only in the epididymis and, Eppin 3 only in the testis were also considered in immunocontraception Eppin is one of several serine-protease that are encoded by genes on human chromosome 20. (4,5). Recently,researchers have been cloned these epididymal protease inhibitors in human and mice. Eppin is involved in sperm maturation and fertilization,and the innate immune system of human epididymis. Immunocontraception with Eppin seems effective and reliable, but its safety need to be further proved(6) Antibodies to Eppin in immunized male monkeys provide an effective and reversible contraception and these antibodies may be effective by interfering with Eppin's interaction with semenogelin during ejaculation. Hydrolysis of semenogelin was performed by prostate specific antigen(7,8). Immunocontraception and, in particular the targeting of antibodies to gamete-specific antigens implicated in sperm egg binding and fertilization, offers an attractive approach to control fertility. The antibodies raised against the sperm specific antigens have proved to be extremely effective at reducing sperm-egg interaction in vitro(9). Sperm has been known to be antigenic for more than a century. There is a strong body of evidence that in humans and in other species at least some antibodies that bind to sperm antigen can cause infertility. These antibodies are of interest because can induce infertility,consequently , they have the potential to be developed for contraceptive purposes in humans and also for the control of feral animal populations(10). In addition, epidemiologic studies indicated that some infertile men who were infected with Ureaplasma urealyticum(UU) displayed positive antisperm antibodies in their serum and/or semen.The existence of cross-reactive antigens(61,50 ,25kDa) between UU and human sperm membrane proteins was confirmed. In fact, a pentapeptide identity(IERLT) was found in anti-rUreG and in antiserum against the synthetic peptide NASP 393-408 and its presence inhibited mouse sperm egg binding and fusion. After immunization by rUreG or the synthetic peptide,81.2 and 75% female mice became sterile, respectively. Besides, the effect on fertility in mice immunized with the synthetic peptide was reversible (11,12) .A recombinant ovalbumin –luteinizing hormone –releasing hormone(ova-LHRH) antigen has been developed for immunocontraception .This vaccine seems an effective immunostimolant for LHRH immunization and contraception(13). Currently,interest was devoted to sperm-reactive human single chain variable fragment (scFv)antibodies. These antibodies seem to offer an available prospective in human sperm function inhibition(14).At the present time,the studies are focused on increasing the immunogenicity and efficacy of the birth control vaccine. A licit suspect consent to hypotisize that the vaccines may be abused by health advocates in developing countries and by their use in vulnerable groups of population.

REFERENCES

[1] Dirnhofer, S., Wick, G., Berger, P. (1995). The suitability of human chorionic gonadotropin (h-CG)-based birth-control vaccines. *Immunol Today*,15(10),469-74.

[2] Jones, W.R. (2005).Vaccination for contraception. Aust.N.Z.J.Obstet. Gynecol. 1994;34(3), 320-9. 3)Naz RK Contraceptive vaccines. *Drugs*,65(5),593-603.

[3] Clauss, A., Lilja, H., Lundwall, A. (2002). A locus on human chromosome 20 contains several genes expressing protease inhibitor domains with homology to whey acid protein. *Biochem.J*, 368(1), 233-42

[4] Guo, X.Q.,Wang, R.J. (2005). Advances in the study of epididymal protease inhibitor. *Zhonghua Nan.Ke Xue*,11(11),851-3.)

[5] Richardson, R.T., Sivashanmugan, P., Hall, S.H., Hamil, K.G., Moore, P.A., Ruben, S.M,, French, F.S., O' Rand, M. (2001).Cloning and sequencing of human Eppin :a novel family of protease inhibitors expressed in the epididymis and testis. *Gene*, 270(1-2),93-102
[6] O'Rand, M.G.,Widgren, E.E.,Wang, Z., Richardson, R.T. (2007).Eppin: an epididymal protease inhibitor and a target for male contraception. Soc.Reprod.Fertil.Suppl. 2007;63:445-53. 8)Wang Z,Widgren EE,Richardson RT,Orand MG. Eppin:a molecular strategy for male contraception. *Soc.Reprod.Fertil. Suppl*, 65, 535-42.
[7] 9)Suri, A. (2004). Sperm specific proteins-potential candidate molecules for fertility control. *Reprod.Biol.Endocrinol*, 2,10.
[8] 10)Chamley, L.W.,Clarke, G.N. (2007).Antisperm antibodies and conception. *Semin. Immunopathol*, 29(2),169-84.
[9] 11)Wiley, C.A., Quinn, P.A. (1984).Enzyme-linked immunosorbent assay for detection of specific antibodies to Ureaplasma urealyticum serotypes. *J.Clin.Microbiol*,19(3), 421-6.
[10] 12)Shi, J.,Yang, Z.,Wang, M.,Cheng, G., Li, D.,Wang, Y., Zhou, Y., Liu, X., Xu, C. (2007). Screening of an antigen target for immunocontraceptives from cross-reactive antigens between human sperm and Ureaplasma urealyticum. *Infect.Immun*, 75(4), 2004-11.
[11] 13)Conforti, V.A., De Avila, D.M.,Cumming, N.S.,Wells, K.J.,Ulker, H.,Reeves, J.J. (2007).The effectiveness of a CpC motif-based adjuvant (CpG ODN 2006) for LHRH immunization.*Vaccine*, 25(35), 6537-43.
[12] 14)Samuel, A.S., Naz, R.K. (2008).Isolation of human single chain variable fragment antibodies against specific sperm antigens for immunocontraceptive development.*Hum.Reprod*,23(6),1324-37.

PROGESTERONE RECEPTOR MODULATORS (PMRS) AND PROGESTERONE ANTAGONISTS (PAS)

Since the discovery of mifepristone (RU 486),other antiprogestins have been synthesized as onapristone(ZK 98.299) and lilopristone(ZK 98.734) which compete with progesterone at the receptor level. These compounds are grouped in the large family of progesterone receptors ligands that include pure progesterone antagonists(PAs)and progesterone receptor modulators (PMRs) (1).Selective progesterone receptor modulators(SPRMs) have mixed agonist-antagonist properties. Antiprogestins can modulate estrogenic effects in various estrogen-dependent tissues.Their complex modulatory effects depend on species,tissues,type of compound,dose and duration of treatment (2)A high dose of mifepristone,200mg administered immediately following ovulation,is highly effective in preventing implantation; however,this antiprogestin is generally used to terminate pregnancy of less than 9 weeks duration.The contraceptive potential of the antiprogestins has been evaluated in clinical and experimental studies.Some of these formulations have partial agonist activity which is mediated primarily through the N-domain of the B-isoform of progesterone receptors(PR),although the mechanism has not yet been defined(3).Both, PMRs as well as PAs have proven antiproliferative effects on endometrium due to interaction with its mitotic activity ,in a dose-dependent manner(2).These effects are endometrium-specific,since the estrogenic effects in the oviduct and vagina are not inhibited by PAs. Administration of antiprogestins such as mifepristone and onapristone ,during the follicular phase of the menstrual cycle, postpones the estrogen rise and the luteinising hormone surge and delays endometrial maturation(4). Studies in animal model reported that anovulation and luteal insufficiency may occur during prolonged treatment(5). As long as treatment is continued ,follicular development is delayed or arrested and ovulation inhibited.Because of anovulation,there may be an unopposed estrogen effect on the endometrium,although this risk may be mitigated by noncompetitive anti-estrogenic activity exhibited by both PAs and PRMs.(6). Interestingly, the treatment with these products is not associated with hypo-estrogenism and bone loss(1).It is assumed that this inhibitory effect of antiprogestins on ovulation is mediated by a blocking effect of progesterone on the pituitary level. Intermittent administration of mifepristone,together with periodic administration of a gestagen,both inhibit ovulation and induce regular withdrawal bleeding. Low weekly,2,5 mg to 5 mg ,and daily doses,0,5mg ,of mifepristone which do not inhibit ovulation ,retard endometrium maturation indicating its strong sensitivity to these compounds (6,7).In contrast,when mifepristone is administered every month, at the end of the cycle ,either alone or together with prostaglandins,it is not very effective in preventing pregnancy(6).Some PRMs have potential use in women with dysfunctional uterine bleeding because of their antiproliferative effects(4) .Chronic, low dose PAs treatment may provide a new option for women who wish to suppress their menstrual periods inducing reversible amenorrhoea (8). In humans, chronic administration of high doses of antiprogestins has, on rare occasions, been associated with endometrial hyperplasia ,presumably a consequence of unopposed estrogen activity.This does not occur with low-doses(9).Intrauterine devices (IUDs) that release progestins are highly effective contraceptives, but they induce breakthrough bleeding that some women find unacceptable. Because progesterone antagonists (APs)are known to suppress the endometrium, induce amenorrhea and inhibit fertility, AP-releasing IUDs (AP-IUDs)has been experimented in macaques. AP-IUD may provide an effective contraception that also controls endometrial bleeding. In fact, it (ZK 230 211) induced in macaques extended, frank menstruation ,when inserted during the late luteal phase, an indication of local APs action. Over time, endometrial glandular and arterial proliferation were inhibited, steroid receptors were elevated, spiral arteries showed degenerative changes, progesterone withdrawal bleeding was prevented, and estradiol-dependent proliferation was suppressed by the AP-IUDs.In conclusion,AP-IUDs suppressed the effects of progesterone on endometrial development and blocked the effects of estrogen on endometrial proliferation, as previously showed for systemic treatment with APs. Therefore, AP IUDs may provide novel contraceptive devices with minimal breakthrough bleeding (10). Modulation of endometrial receptivity is a promising approach for fertility regulation since it allows a contraceptive to act specifically at the endometrium. This was corroborated by previous observations that treatment with low doses of a pure progesterone antagonist (PA, antiprogestin), onapristone (ZK 98.299), in bonnet monkeys inhibited fertility by selectively retarding endometrial development, without affecting the hypophyseal-hypothalamic function.(11).Hence,the properties of PAs and PRMs open up new applications in contraceptive strategies introducing the new concept of "Endometrial Contraception".

REFERENCES

[1] Chabbert-Buffet, N., Meduri, G., Bouchard, P., Spitz, I.M. (2005).Selective progesterone receptor modulators and progesterone antagonists:mechanisms of action and clinical applications.*Hum.Reprod.Update,* 11(3),293-307.
[2] Chwalisz, K., Brenner, R.M., Fuhrmann, U.U., Hess-Stumpp, H., Elger, W. (2000).Antiproliferative effects of progesterone antagonists and progesteron e receptor modulators on the endometrium.*Steroids*,65(10-11),741-51.
[3] Wardell, S.E., Edwards, D.P. (2005).Mechanisms controlling agonist and antagonist potential of selective progesterone receptor modulators(SPRMs).*Semin.Reprod.Med*,23(1), 9-21.
[4] Spitz, I.M., Chwalisz, K. (2000). Progesterone receptor modulators and progesterone antagonists in women's health.*Steroids*,65,807-15.
[5] Katkam, R.R.,Gopalkrishnan, K.,Chwalisz, K., Schillinger, E., Puri, C.P. (1995). Onapristone(ZK 98.299):a potential antiprogestin for endometrial contraception. *Am.J.Obstet.Gynecol*,173(3),779-87.

[6] Spitz, I.M., Van Look, P.F.,Coelingh Bennink, H.J. (2000).The use of progesterone antagonists and progesterone receptor modulators in contraception.*Steroids,*65(10-11),817-23.
[7] Bygdeman, M., Danielsson, K.G., Swahn, M.L. (1907).The possible use of antiprogestins for contraception.*Acta Obstet.Gynecol.Scand.Suppl*, 164,75-7.
[8] Slayden, O.D.,Chwalisz, K., Brenner, R.M. (2001).Reversible suppression of menstruation with progesterone antagonists in rhesus macaques. *Human Reprod*,16(8),1562-74.
[9] Spitz, I.M., Robbins, A. (1990).Mechanism of action and clinical effects of progestins on the non-pregnant uterus.*Hum.Reprod.Update*,4(5),584-93.
[10] Nayak, N.R., Slayden, O.D., Mah, K.,Chwalisz, K., Brenner, R.M. (2007).Antiprogestin-releasing intrauterine devices: a novel approach to endometrial contraception.*Contraception*,75(6), S104-11.
[11] Puri, C.P., Katkam, R.R., Sachdeva, G., Patil, V., Manjramkar, D.D., Kholkute, S.D. (2000).Endometrial contraception: modulation of molecular determinants of uterine receptivity. *Steroids*,65(10-11),783-94.

CONTRACEPTIVE COUNSELING

The choice of the contraceptive method takes into account the contraindications of the method as well as the patient's personnel history,the type of demand,the needs and the fears. In fact,observance requires proper information and reassurance on side effects, particularly on menstruation disorders to avoid drop out.Instructions need to be clear and given in the language that the patient can understand. It helps to have written material to give to the patient.Until now,we have limited evidence about what works to help users choose an appropriate contraceptive method(1).Therefore, despite the high effectiveness, hormonal contraceptives report difficulty in adherence regimen and low rates for long-term continuation. However,there is a definite increase in contraceptive uptake in women provided with educational leaflets and counselling sessions with a shift toward use of more reliable contraceptive methods(2).Hormonal contraceptives afford much better efficacy in preventing pregnancy when used with full compliance.Unfortunately,also minor effects do contribute to the high discontinuation rates seen(3).One of the best means to improve outcomes is through high-quality gynecologist-woman communication (4).Besides, despite the efficacy of HCs,the missed pill is common and contribute to unwanted pregnancy. For these women nondaily HC-options may be considered: levonorgestrel-5 year intrauterine system, medroxyprogesterone quarterly injection, Lunelle monthly injection,monthly vaginal ring and weekly transdermal patch. Long-acting progestogen-only methods,such as injectable and implantable may be planned for women who need to avoid estrogens. Furthermore, the accuracy of contraceptive counselling is a priority to avoid hazardous prescription as well as to select the method, correspondent to woman's expectation. In fact, almost half of the users who discontinued a contraceptive method were unsatisfied with it(5).Extended or continuous regimens may be appreciated by women who have an intense lifestyle and prefer to avoid menstruation and in those who have recurrent menstrual problems as dysmenorrhea,endometriosis or headache(6,7,8,9). Today,many teenagers are sexually active at earlier ages than in former times,before they are cognitively able to develop a responsible sexual behaviour.Therefore,considering the frequency of their sexual intercourses and the short period of sexual partnerships,effective contraceptive counselling for adolescents should be a priority(10,11).During the vulnerable period of adolescence,decision relating to contraception may occur and dual method (hormonal contraceptive plus condom)may be advisable(12). When possible,the involvement of the mother can support the girl's decision and to give more information regarding eventual previous illness or genetic anomalies, particularly if related to coagulation system(Leiden factor mutation,deficit of protein C,S,factorVII or VIII ..) (13). Besides,we believe that teens' knowledge about the contraceptive and noncontraceptive benefits might motivate more consistent pill taking,and the involvement of their mother must encourage its regular use(14).In adolescents,depot medroxyprogesterone may be an ideal option, but its use is associated with poor continuation rates. Although the major problem is menstrual irregularity;the time,expense and inconvenience of a gynaecological visit also pose a barrier to use.Self-administration might make visit unnecessary.Adequate training and counselling regarding bleeding patterns may maximize success rates with self-administration (15).

Currently,the need for contraception in a period of life characterized by irregular menstrual cycles as the perimenopause, represents a social event.The introduction of new lower-dose contraceptives and progestin-only formulations as implants and IUD-releasing progestin has deeply changed the indications for hormonal contraception, allowing its use in women in whom it was previously contraindicated(16.17,18,19,20). Although, gynecologist's personal opinions and poor knowledges about this field , often lead to refuse contraception in older women. Other important problems regard the contraceptive counselling post-abortion,post-partum and the contraceptive guidance for women at risk of sexually transmitted diseases or affected by HPV, and/or HIV infections

(21,22,23,24,25,26,27,28,29,30,31). Although many studies have shown a disappointing periabortion contraceptive uptake; it was found that contraceptive counseling by a dedicate team, during pre-abortion visit, can dramatically improve post-abortion contraception uptake. In addition, according to the woman's preference it is possible to provide immediate post-abortal IUD-insertion (32,33).Preconception counselling is very important in adolescent sexually active with type 1-diabetes.In fact,early and unsafe sexual practices may increase their risk for unplanned pregnancy that could result in pregnancy-related complications. Enhancing knowledge and attitude towards preconception counselling and reproductive health education may reduce these risks and may permit a future,healthy reproductive life(34,35,36).Expert counselling is necessary to plan birth control strategy in women affected by chronic serious diseases or transplant-recipients.In these women,sometimes there is difficulty to select a hormonal contraceptive risk-free, but pregnancy may be even riskier(37,38,39,40,41,42). Therapy selection should be individualized and based on the patient's specific needs and global related health risks.Clearly,for the management of these cases and the individual risk evaluation,specific competence is necessary about each particular pathologic entity and the possible contraceptive action.In fact, the superficial evaluation can lead to refuse a safe contraceptive method when suitable, or to prescribe a hormonal contraceptive when hazardous. Adherence and continuation are fundamentally important to the successful use of hormonal contraception(43,44).Expert and accurate counselling can help women to achieve adequate informations ,choosing the contraceptive method corresponding to their expectations.We believe that this patient procedure might motivate more consistent contraceptive taking and encourage its regular use(12,14).

REFERENCES

[1] Lopez, L.M., Steiner, M.J.,Grimes, D.A.,Schulz, K.F. (2008). Strategies for communicating contraceptive effectiveness. *Cochrane Database Syst.Rev*,2,CD006964.
[2] Tafelski, T., Boehm, K.E. (1995).Contraception in the adolescent patient.*Prim.Care*,22(1),145-59.
[3] Saeed, G.A., Fakhar, S., Rahim, F.,Tabassum, S. (2008).Change in trend of contraceptive uptake-effect of educational leaflets and counselling. *Contraception*,77(5), 377-81.
[4] Dominguez, C.E. (2007). Patient counseling women using oral contraceptives.*Manag.Care Interface*, 20(6),33-7.

[5]   Moreau, C., Cleland, K.,Trussel, J. (2007).Contraceptive discontinuation attribuited to method dissatisfaction in the United States. *Contraception,*76(4), 267-72.
[6]   Freeman, S. (2004). Nondaily hormonal contraception: considerations in contraceptive choice and patient counseling. *J.Am.Acad.Nurse Pract*, 16(6), 226-38
[7]   Nelson, A.L. (2007). Communicating with patients about extended-cycle and continuous use of oral contraceptives. *J.Womens Health*,16(4), 463-70.
[8]   Hitchcock, C.L., Prior, J.C. (2004).Evidence about extending the duration of oral contraceptive use to suppress menstruation. *Women Health Issues*,14(6), 201-11.
[9]   Edelman, A.B.,Gallo, M.F., Jensen, J.T.,Nichols, M.D.,Schulz, K.F.,Grimes, D.A. (2005).Continuous or extended cycle vs.cyclic use of combined oral contraceptives for contraception. *Cochrane Database Syst. Rev*,20(3),CD004695
[10] Santelli, J.S.,Morrow, B., Anderson, J.E.,Lindberg, L.D. (2006). Contraceptive use and pregnancy among U.S. high school students,1991-2003.Pespect.*Sex Reprod.Health*,38,106-11.
[11] Anderson, J.E., Santelli, J.S.,Morrow, B. (2006).Trends in adolescent contraceptive use: unprotected and poorly protected sex,1991-2003.J.Adolesc.*Health*,38,734-9.
[12] Rove, C.,Perlmutter Silverman, P., Krauss, B. (2007).A brief,low-cost,theory-based intervention to promote dual method use by black and Latina female adolescents:a randomized clinical trial. *Health Educ.Behav*,34(4),608-21.
[13] Ornstein, R.M., Fisher, M.M. (2006). Hormonal contraception in adolescents:special considerations.Paediatr. *Drugs*, 8(1), 25-45.
[14] Sabatini R.,Orsini, G.,Cagiano, R., Loverro, G. (2007). Noncontraceptive benefits of two combined oral contraceptives with antiandrogenic properties among adolescents. *Contraception*,76, 342-347.
[15] Prabhakaran, S. (2008). Self-administration of injectable contraceptives.*Contraception*, 77 (5),315-7.
[16] Kailas,N.A.,Sifakis, S.,Koumantakis, E. (2005). Contraception durin perimenopause.*Eur. J.Contracept Reprod.Health Care,*10(1), 19-25.
[17] Bathema, R. K., Guillebaud, J. (2006). Contraception for the older woman: an up date. *Climacteric*,9(4), 264-76.
[18] Thorneycroft, I.H. (1993).Contraception in women older than 40 years of age. *Obstet. Gynecol. Clin. North. Am*,20(2), 273-8

[19] Shaaban, M.M. (1996).The perimenopause and contraception. *Maturitas*,23(2),181-92.
[20] Speroff L, Sulak PJ. (1995).Contraception in the later reproductive years:a valid aspect of preventive health care. *Dialogues Contracept*,4(5), 1-4
[21] Fasubaa, O.B., Ojo, O.D. (2004). Impact of post-abortion counselling in a semi-urban town of Western Nigeria. *J.Obstet.Gynaecol*, 24(3),298-303.
[22] Engin-Ustun, Y.,Ustun, Y.,Cetin, F.,Meydanli, M.M.,Kafkasli, A.,Sezgin, B. (2007). Effect of postpartum counseling on postpartum contraceptive use.*Arch.Gynecol.Obstet*,275(6), 429-32.
[23] Bulut, A.,Turan, J.M. (1995). Postpartum family planning and health needs of women of low income in Istambul.*Stud.Fam.Plann*,26(2), 88-100.
[24] Nùnez-Urquiza, R.M.,Hernandez-Prado, B.,Garcia-Barrios, C.,Gonzàlez, D.,Walker, D. (2003). Unwanted adolescent pregnancy and post-partum utilization of contraceptive methods. *Salud.Publica Mex,*45(1), S 92-102.
[25] Kjos, S.L. (2007).After pregnancy complicated by diabetes:postpartum care and education. *Obstet.Gynecol.Clin.North Am*,34(2), 335-49.
[26] De Villiers, E.M. (2003).Relationship between steroid hormone contraceptives and HPV, cervical intraepithelial neoplasia and cervical carcinoma. *Int.J.Cancer*,103(6), 70
[27] Moodley, M.,Moodley, J.,Chetty, R.,Herrington, C.S. (2003).The role of steroid contraceptive hormones in the pathogenesis of invasive cervical cancer:a review. *Int.J.Gynecol.Cancer*,13(2), 103-10
[28] Green, J., Berrington deGonzales, A., Smith, J.S., Mfranceschi, S.,Appleby, P., Plummer, M., Beral, V. (2003).Human papillomavirus and use of oral contraceptives.*Br.J.Cancer*,88(11),1713-20.
[29] Aaron, E.,Levine, A.B. (2005).Gynecologic care and family planning for HIV-infected women. *AIDS Read*,15(8),420-3,426-8.
[30] Delvaux, T., Noslinger, C. (2007). Reproductive choice for women and men living with HIV: contraception, abortion and fertility.*Reprod.Health Matters*,15(29 Suppl.),46-66.
[31] Mitchell, H.S., Stephens, E. (2004). Contraception choice for HIV positive women. *Sex.Transm.Infect*, 80(3),167-73.
[32] Yassin, A.S.,Cordwell, D. (2005). Does dedicated pre-abortion contraception counselling help to improve post-abortion contraception uptake? *J.Fam.Plann.Reprod.HealthCare*,31(2),115-6.
[33] El-Tagy, A., Sakr, E., Sokal, D.C.,Issa, A.H. (2003). Safety and acceptability of post-abrtal IUD insertion and the importance of counselling.*Contraception*, 67(3),229-34.

[34] Klinke, J.,Toth, E.L. (2003). Preconception care for women with type 1 diabetes. *Can.Fam.Physician*, 49,769-73.
[35] Charron-Prochownik, D.,Sereika, S.M.,Wang, S.L.,Hannan, M.F., Fischi, A.R.,Stewart, S.H., Dean – McElhinny, T. (2006).Reproductive health and preconception counseling awareness in adolescents with diabetes:what they don't know can hurt them.*Diabetes Educ*,32(2),235-42.
[36] Charron-Prochownik, D., Ferons-Hannan, M., Sereika, S.,Becker, D. (2008).*Randomize Efficacy Trial of Early Preconception Counseling FOE Diabetic Teens (READY –Girls)Diabetes Care*,Apr. 14.(Epub. Ahead of print).
[37] Teal, S.B.,Ginosar, D.M. (2007).Contraception for women with chronic medical conditions. *Obstet.Gynecol.Clin.North Am,* 34(1),113-26.
[38] Shilling, M.K., Zimmermann, A., Radaelli, C., Seiler, C.A., Buchler, M.W. (2000).Liver nodules resembling focal nodular hyperplasia after hepatic venous thrombosis. *J.Hepatol*,33(4),673-6.
[39] Shortell, C.K., Schwartz. S.I. (1991). Hepatic adenoma and focal nodular hyperplasia.Surg. Gynecol. Obstet, 173(5), 426-31.
[40] Lakasing, L., Khamashta, M. (2001).Contraceptive practices in women with systemic lupus erythematous and/or antiphospholipid syndrome:what advice should we be giving? *J.Fam. Plann.Reprod.Health Care*, 27(1), 7-12
[41] Seifert-Klauss, V., Kaemmerer, H., Brunner, B., Schneider, K.T., Hess, J. (2000).Contraception in patients with congenital heart defects. *Z.Kardiol*,89(7),606-11.
[42] Rongières-Bertrand, C., Fernandez, H. (1998).Contraceptive use in female transplant recipients. *Contracept.Fertil.Sex*, 26(2),845-50.
[43] Dominguez, C.E. (2007). Patient counseling women using oral contraceptives.*Manag.Care Interface,* 20(6),33-7.
[44] Halpern, V.,Grimes, D.A.,Lopez, L.,Gallo, M.F. (2006).Strategies to improve adherence acceptability of hormonal methods for contraception. *Cochrane Database Syst. Rev*,25(1), CD004317.

CONCLUSION

The world population is expected to increase by 2.6 billion to 9.1 billion in 2050 (1). Particularly, the developing countries contribute to this growth with consequent increase of their social and economic problems .So,this overpopulation stresses the discrepancy between developed and developing states. The report "The Evolution of the Family in Europe 2008" declares that over 1.16

milion of legal abortions are performed each year in Europe. The real global incidence is unknown and each supposed percentage results underestimated.Besides,an estimated 19 million unsafe abortions occur worldwide each year,resulting in the death of about 70,000 women.The majority of these abortion occur in under-resourced settings as sub-Saharan Africa,Central and Southeast Asia,and Latin America and the Caribbean.The causes include inadequate delivery systems for contraception,restrictive abortion laws, cultural and religious influences(2,3,4).With worldwide unintended pregnancy rates approaching 50% of all pregnancies,there is an increased need for the improvement of hormonal contraception acceptability,compliance and continuation.Currently,pharmacological methods of contraception are reversible contraceptive steroids formulated in pills,patches, intravaginal rings, subdermal implants and injections(5,6). Despite the safety profile of current COCs, fears of adverse metabolic and vascular effects caused by estrogen component, and possible neoplastic effects of these formulations remain.Misperceptions and concerns about side-effects,especially those affecting the menstrual cycle and increased body weight ,are often given as reason for discontinuation.However, these disorders are not clinically significant.They can lead to erratic method use or even to discontinuation(7).Much of the woman's dissatisfaction because of menstrual changes can be averted by careful counselling prior to method prescription. Open dialogue explaining the potential for bleeding irregularities is crucial in this time, in order to avoid the discontinuation that places the woman at risk of unwilling pregnancy.The hormonal contraceptive prescription in some women at risk might be considered a hazard, but an expert individualized evaluation of gynecologist may consent it. Most women with congenital cardiac disease can safely use oral contraceptives,especially low-estrogen combinations or progestin-only preparations(8).

Clearly, oral contraceptives should be avoided in all patients at particular risk of thromboembolic complications because of pulmonary hypertension, Eisenmenger syndrome, rhythm disturbances, reduced ventricular function,arterial hypertension, infectious complications (endocarditis) or hyperlipidemia. Intrauterine devices-releasing progestin which are very effective, have no metabolic side effects and merely carry a small risk of endocarditis(9). Other medical conditions require our attention.During hormonal contraceptive use,some cases of subhepatic vein thrombosis or the Budd-Chiari syndrome, associated to focal nodular hyperplasia as well as adenoma have been reported(10,11) In the meantime,it is mandatory to avoid combined hormonal contraception in SLE patients with high levels of antiphospholipid antibodies and, in those with active nephritis(12,13). In fact, these women, when use combined oral contraceptives are at high risk of thromboses (St.Thomas'Hospital-London) (12,13). Progress in the area of female reproduction is showing great promise for identifying new contraceptives drug targets (14). Today,,the properties of Selective progesterone receptor modulators (PRMs) and progesterone antagonists(PAs) open up new applications in contraceptive strategies introducing the new concept of "Endometrial Contraception"(15). In the meantime,there is necessity to develop newer,possibly nonsteroidal and non hormonal contraceptives.Recent advancements in our understanding of ovarian endocrinology,coupled with molecular biology and transgenic technology,have enabled identification of several factors that are functionally critical in the regulation of female fertility. Large investments are being made focalized on prevention of unwilling pregnancy and sexually transmitted disease in several countries, but the relevance of the problem requires the interest at international political levels. Contraception is a crucial human right for its role in health,development and quality of life.In spite of shortcomings of currently available male contraception,1/3 of the couples that use contraception worldwide rely on male methods, suggesting that the development of a safe,effective,reversible and affordable contraceptive method for men would meet a critical need(16).Because rates of unintended pregnancy,abortion and unintended birth are very high among adult women in the United States,it is important to identify interventions that can increase contraceptive use in the population, such as vaccines.Currently, vaccines are still experimental and until now were tested in animal and in women of developing countries(17,18).A research plan that rigorously assesses the impact of different approaches to increasing contraceptive use among adult and young women, should be an integral part of any long-term effort to prevent unintended pregnancy (19)

REFERENCES

[1] Erkkola, R. (2006). Recent advances in contraception. *Minerva Ginecol,* 58(4), 295-305.
[2] Grimes, D.A. (2003).Unsafe abortion:the silent scourge.*Br.Med.Bull*, 67, 99-113.
[3] Okonofua,F.(2006).Abortion and maternal mortality in the developing world. *J.Obstet.Gynaecol.Can*, 28(11),974-9.
[4] Fawcus,S.R. (2008). Maternal mortality and unsafe abortion.*BestPract.Res.Clin.Obstet.Gynaecol*, 22(3), 533-48.

[5] Economidis, M.A., Mishell, D.R. Jr. (2005).Pharmacological female contraception: an overview of past and future use.Expert Opin.*Invastig.Drugs*, 14(4), 449-56.
[6] Benagiano, G.,Bastianelli, C., Farris, M. Contraception today. Ann.N.Y.Acad.Sci.2006; 1092;1-32.
[7] Cheung, E., Free, C. (2005). Factors influencing young women's decision-making regarding hormonal contraceptives: a qualitative study.*Contraception*, 71, 426-31.
[8])Seifert-Klauss, V., Kaemmerer, H., Brunner, B., Schneider, K.T., Hess, J. (2000).Contraception in patients with congenital heart defects.*Z.Kardiol*, 89(7), 606-11.
[9] Teal, S.B.,Ginosar, D.M. (2007).Contraception for women with chronic medical conditions.*Obstet.Gynecol.Clin.North Am*,34(1), 113- 26.
[10] Tong, H.K., Fai, G.L., Ann, L.T., Hock, O.B. (1981).Budd-Chiari syndrome and hepatic adenomas associated with oral contraceptives.A case report. *Singapore Med.J,* 22(3),168-72.
[11] Shilling, M.K., Zimmermann, A., Radaelli, C., Seiler, C.A., Buchler, M.W. (2000).Liver nodules resembling focal nodular hyperplasia after hepatic venous thrombosis.*J.Hepatol*, 33(4),673-6.
[12] Jungers, P., Dougados, M., Pèlissier, C., Kuttenn, F., Tron, F., Pertuiset, N., Bach, J.F. (1982). Effect of hormonal contraception on the course of lupus nephropathy.Nouv.*Presse Med*, 11(51), 3765-8.
[13] Lakasing, L., Khamashta, M. (2001).Contraceptive practices in women with systemic lupus erythematous and/or antiphospholipid syndrome :what advice should we be giving? *J.Fam. Plann.Reprod.Health Care*, 27(1), 7-12.
[14] Chengalvala, M.V., Meade, E.H. Jr, Cottom, J.E., Hoffman, W.H., Shanno, L.K.,Wu, M.M., Kopf, G.S., Shen, E.S. (2006).Regulation of female fertility and identification of future contraceptive targets.*Curr. Pharm. Des*,12(30), 3915-28.
[15] Chabbert-Buffet, N., Meduri, G., Bouchard, P., Spitz, I.M. (2005). Selective progesterone receptor modulators and progesterone antagonists:mechanisms of action and clinical applications.*Hum.Reprod.Update*, 11(3), 293-307.
[16] Costantino, A.,Cerpolini, S., Perrone, A.M.,Ghi, T., Pelusi, C., Pelusi, G., Meriggiola, M.C. (2007).Current status and future perspectives in male contraception.*Minerva Ginecol*, 59(3), 299-310.
[17] Suri, A. (2004). Sperm specific proteins-potential candidate molecules for fertility control.*Reprod.Biol. Endocrinol*, 2,10.

[18] Chamley, L.W., Clarke, G.N. (2007).Antisperm antibodies and conception.*Semin.Immunopathol*, 29 (2),169-84
[19] Kirby, D. (2008).The impact of programs to increase contraceptive use among adult women:a review of experimental and quasi-experimental studies.*Perspect Sex Reprod Health. Mar*, 40(1),34-41.

INDEX

A

abdominal, 25, 26, 50, 60, 75
abnormalities, 2, 39
abortion, 34, 41, 48, 49, 74, 114, 117, 119, 120
absorption, 62
acceptors, 94
access, 40
accidents, vii, 6, 10, 27
accuracy, 114
acetate, viii, 8, 11, 34, 47, 49, 59, 62, 67, 72, 78, 83, 86, 88, 90, 91, 94, 102, 103
acid, 59, 62, 75, 86, 109
acne, viii, 44, 86, 88, 97
acne vulgaris, 86
activation, 30
acute, 5, 7, 14, 27, 29, 59, 63, 81, 87, 89
acute intermittent porphyria, 59, 63, 87, 89
Adams, 50, 89
adaptation, 101
adenocarcinoma, 38, 40, 51
adenoma, 41, 44, 56, 57, 58, 64, 77, 118, 119
adenomas, 41, 44, 56, 57, 58, 60, 76, 121
administration, viii, 15, 42, 61, 90, 107, 111, 114, 116
adolescence, 114
adolescent female, 84, 90, 94
adolescent patients, 81
adolescents, ix, xi, 40, 53, 73, 78, 82, 84, 88, 91, 93, 94, 97, 103, 114, 116, 118
adult, 11, 120, 122
adults, 71
adverse event, 93
aetiology, 25, 26
age, ix, xi, 1, 3, 5, 6, 8, 10, 11, 12, 13, 22, 34, 35, 39, 41, 43, 44, 46, 47, 48, 65, 83, 85, 87, 92, 116
agents, 15, 44, 56, 82, 86
aging, ix
agonist, 110, 112
AIDS, 66, 71, 73, 117
albumin, 12, 22, 65
aldosterone, 13, 23
allergic, 30, 87, 89
allergic reaction, 87, 89
allergy, 30, 31, 86
allograft, 67, 68
allograft survival, 68
alpha, 75, 78
alternative, viii, 7, 26, 39, 62, 81, 88
alternatives, 108
amenorrhea, 111
amplitude, 101
Amsterdam, xi
anabolic, 45
analgesics, 88
anaphylaxis, 86, 87, 88, 89, 90
ANCA, 30
androgen, ix, 22, 43, 45, 86, 88, 104

androgen receptors, ix, 43, 45
androgens, ix, 42, 43, 45
angioedema, 25, 26, 86, 87, 89
angioneurotic edema, 26
angiotensin, 13, 22
animals, 28, 108
anorexia, 75
antagonist, 9, 110, 112
antagonists, 110, 112, 113, 120, 121
antibiotics, 106
Antibodies, 108
antibody, 15, 30, 86, 89, 108
anticoagulant, 9, 60
anticoagulants, 19
anticonvulsant, 62
anti-estrogenic, 111
antigen, 30, 37, 109, 110
antihypertensive drugs, 70
anti-inflammatory, 42
antiphospholipid, 63, 66, 86, 89, 118, 119, 121
antiphospholipid antibodies, 63, 119
antiphospholipid syndrome, 66, 118, 121
antiretroviral, 63, 67
antiretrovirals, 67
antiserum, 109
antithrombin, 8, 19, 61, 65
anxiety, 101
anxiety disorder, 101
APC, 9, 20, 60
apoptosis, 43, 47, 49, 59
application, 35
arousal, ix
arterial hypertension, 61, 69, 70, 119
arteries, 7, 9, 29, 112
arterioles, 29
arteriovenous malformation, 5, 60
artery, 6, 18, 27, 28, 29
ascites, 27
assessment, 34, 94, 102
associations, ix, 34, 39, 42, 46, 48
asthenia, 75
asthma, 30, 31
asymptomatic, 19, 76, 105, 106
atherosclerosis, 3, 6, 17

atopy, 30
atrophy, 38
attacks, 5, 17, 25, 26, 59, 63, 84, 89
attention, 39, 119
atypical, 38, 51, 87
aura, 5, 17, 61, 85
Australia, 55
autoimmune, 30, 87, 90, 108
autoimmune disease, 30
autosomal dominant, 25, 37
availability, 11
awareness, 79, 82, 84, 118

B

bacilli, 106
barrier, 39, 62, 72, 106, 114
basal cell carcinoma, 56
bcl-2, 47, 59
behavior, 105
beneficial effect, 10, 33
benefits, xi, 42, 51, 85, 88, 93, 97, 114, 116
benign, 35, 43, 44, 45, 50, 63, 76, 85
benign tumors, 44, 45
beta, 108
bias, 2, 49, 102
bilateral, 35
bile, 76
binding, 62, 108
binding globulin, 62
biochemical, xii, 18, 68
biochemistry, 86
biological, vii, 101, 103
biology, 48
Biomarker, xi, 48
biopsy, 30, 38, 87
birth, vii, 41, 43, 46, 47, 70, 72, 75, 79, 104, 105, 109, 115, 120
birth control, vii, 70, 72, 79, 104, 105, 109, 115
births, 37, 46
black, 73, 116
bladder, 47, 59
bladder cancer, 47, 59
blastocyst, 107

bleeding, vii, 5, 28, 35, 39, 62, 92, 95, 96, 97, 98, 111, 114, 119
blindness, 27
blood, ix, 2, 7, 9, 12, 14, 20, 22, 23, 26, 61, 65, 68, 80, 82
blood flow, 7, 9
blood group, 20
blood pressure, ix, xi, 2, 7, 12, 13, 14, 22, 23, 61, 65, 68, 82
body composition, 91, 93
body image, 91
body mass index (BMI), 8, 14, 37, 42, 68
body weight, ix, 23, 91, 93, 119
bone, 27, 62, 92, 94, 111
bone density, 92
bone loss, 111
bone marrow, 27
Bone mineral density, 94
brain, 101
Brazil, 94
Brazilian, 92
BRCA, viii, xi, 34, 51
BRCA1, xi, 34, 35, 37, 48, 49, 50
BRCA2, xi, 34, 37, 48, 49, 50
breakdown, 62
breast, viii, xi, 33, 34, 37, 48, 49, 50, 51, 53, 91
breast cancer, viii, xi, 33, 34, 37, 48, 49, 50, 51
bronchial asthma, 30
Budd-Chiari syndrome, 45, 58, 60, 65, 75, 76, 119, 121

C

calcium, 62
cancer, xi, 33, 34, 36, 37, 38, 39, 41, 43, 44, 45, 46, 47, 48, 49, 50, 51, 52, 53, 54, 55, 57, 58, 59, 66, 117
cancer cells, 35
cancer screening, 40, 53
cancerous cells, 34
cancers, 33, 35, 36, 40, 41, 49, 51
Candida, 87, 90, 105, 106, 107
candidates, 37

candidiasis, 105, 106, 107
capacitance, 7, 9
capacity, 62
Cape Town, 63, 89
carbohydrate, 10, 70, 77, 81, 82, 83
carbohydrate metabolism, 10, 79, 81, 82, 83
carcinogenesis, 36, 39, 42
carcinogenic, 45
carcinoma, 37, 38, 40, 41, 44, 47, 50, 57, 59, 70
carcinomas, 38, 51
cardiovascular, viii, x, xii, 1, 3, 5, 10, 13, 14, 17, 21, 77, 86
cardiovascular disease, viii, x, 3, 13, 14, 77
cardiovascular risk, 1, 5, 14
Caribbean, 119
carrier, xi, 10, 48
causal interpretation, 34
causal relationship, 60
causation, 50
cavities, 26
CD4, 40, 63, 72
cell, 31, 43, 44, 56, 57, 58, 59
cell cycle, 43
cell growth, 59
central retinal artery occlusion, 28
cerebral function, 4
cerebral venous thrombosis, 64
cerebrovascular, 4
cerebrovascular accident, 5
cervical, 39, 52, 53, 72, 73, 106, 117
cervical cancer, 39, 52, 53, 117
cervical carcinoma, 40, 52, 117
cervical intraepithelial neoplasia, 52, 117
cervicitis, 72
cervix, 52, 53
chemoprevention, 35, 38, 42, 51
chemopreventive, 38
childbearing, ix, 22, 65, 67
children, 27, 43
Chinese, 16
Chinese women, 16
chlamydia, 72
Chlamydia trachomatis, 72
cholecystectomy, 76

cholestasis, 63, 75
cholesterol, vii, 13, 76, 78
chromosome, 108, 109
chronic, 25, 30, 65, 69, 70, 111, 115, 118, 121
cigarette smoke, 3
cigarette smokers, 3
cigarette smoking, 41, 47
cigarettes, 2, 13
circadian, 101
classes, 43
classical, 30
classified, 39
clinical, ix, 11, 14, 22, 29, 33, 36, 40, 45, 63, 64, 65, 73, 75, 79, 94, 102, 106, 108, 111, 112, 113, 116, 121
clinical trial, 73, 102, 108, 116
clinical trials, 102, 108
clinically significant, 80, 95, 119
clinicians, 25
clinicopathologic, 51
clustering, 37
coagulation, 2, 4, 7, 8, 10, 11, 14, 18, 70, 114
coagulation factor, 4, 8, 10
coagulation factors, 10
Cochrane, 83, 98, 115, 116, 118
COCs, vii, ix, 2, 4, 6, 11, 28, 33, 63, 69, 79, 84, 86, 95, 101, 104, 119
cognitive, 101, 102
coherence, 101
cohort, xi, 4, 8, 12, 16, 18, 19, 42, 46, 48, 54, 58, 59, 78, 92, 94
colic, 27, 76
Collaboration, 52
colon, 41, 50, 53, 54
colon cancer, 41, 50, 54
colonization, 87, 90, 105, 107
colorectal, 41, 53, 54
colorectal cancer, 41, 53, 54
combined oral contraceptives, xi, 2, 14, 15, 29, 33, 39, 63, 68, 78, 84, 85, 86, 88, 93, 97, 101, 104, 116, 120
communication, 113
compensation, 11, 81
competence, 115
complement, 30

compliance, viii, ix, 91, 103, 113, 119
complications, 3, 6, 27, 28, 29, 30, 61, 66, 67, 75, 76, 79, 88, 115, 119
components, xii, 21, 22, 62, 72, 101
composition, 76
compounds, 42, 110
concentration, 38, 78
conception, 60, 70, 72, 79, 107, 110, 122
condom, 72, 114
condoms, 104, 105, 106
confounding variables, 8
Congress, iv
consent, 109, 119
contact dermatitis, 88, 90
continuing, 42
contraceptives, vii, ix, x, xi, xii, 3, 4, 6, 8, 11, 12, 14, 16, 17, 18, 20, 21, 22, 23, 25, 27, 28, 29, 31, 33, 34, 36, 38, 39, 41, 43, 44, 47, 48, 49, 50, 51, 52, 54, 55, 57, 58, 59, 60, 63, 64, 65, 66, 67, 68, 69, 70, 72, 75, 77, 82, 83, 84, 85, 86, 90, 91, 93, 94, 97, 98, 99, 100, 101, 102, 103, 104, 105, 106, 111, 113, 114, 116, 117, 120, 121
control, ix, x, 2, 6, 15, 16, 17, 22, 41, 43, 49, 53, 55, 57, 59, 68, 72, 75, 79, 85, 93, 94, 97, 98, 99, 101, 103, 104, 105, 106, 107, 108, 109, 110, 121
control group, 2, 106
controlled, 73, 81, 85, 88, 93, 96, 97
controlled trials, 93
copper, 78, 92, 94, 95
corpus luteum, 107
correlation, ix, 39
correlations, 17, 31
counsel, 70
counseling, 35, 67, 71, 81, 82, 84, 96, 115, 116, 117, 118
couples, ix, 73, 120
creatinine, 68
cross-sectional, 85
C-terminal, 108
cultural, 119
culture, 104
CVD, viii
cycles, 11, 67, 79, 83, 91, 93, 95, 104

cyclosporine, 70
cyproterone acetate, 11
cyst, 99, 100
cystine, 108
cysts, 99, 100
cytochrome, 22, 62

D

danger, 67, 68
death, xii, 2, 10, 14, 21, 25, 63, 119
death rate, 10
deaths, 6, 15, 36
defects, 2, 8, 14, 18, 65, 71, 118, 121
deficiency, xi, 4, 16, 19, 25, 61, 64, 65, 92
deficit, 100, 114
definition, 102
degenerate, 44
degradation, 77
degree, 11, 81
delays, 111
delivery, 68, 70, 119
delta, 59, 75, 86
demand, 113
density, 92, 94
depressed, x
depression, 101, 102, 103
depressive disorder, 101
depressive symptoms, 101, 102
derivatives, viii, 78
dermal, 46
dermatitis, 87, 88, 89, 90
dermatological, 86
dermatology, 88
dermatosis, 89
descending colon, 41
desire, ix, 70, 103, 104
detection, 30, 110
developed countries, ix, 39
developing countries, 109, 118, 120
diabetes, x, xii, 2, 6, 61, 67, 78, 82, 83, 84, 85, 105, 115, 117, 118
diabetes mellitus, xii, 61, 78, 83, 105
diabetic, xii, 80, 83
diagnostic, 30, 85

diagnostic criteria, 85
diastolic pressure, 12, 13
diet, 42
dimer, 9
direct action, 77
disease progression, 63, 66
diseases, ix, x, 6, 12, 17, 25, 30, 81, 115
disorder, 7, 60, 87
disposition, 7
dissatisfaction, 96, 116, 119
distal, 92
distribution, 44
DNA, 37, 43
dosage, 3, 70, 100
dose-response relationship, 14, 65
dosing, 50
down-regulation, 7, 9, 11
draft, 69
drug interaction, 62
drug targets, 120
drug therapy, 70
drugs, 17, 62, 65, 66, 87
Dubin-Johnson syndrome, 63, 76
duration, 2, 6, 10, 34, 37, 39, 41, 43, 44, 47, 51, 75, 76, 84, 87, 92, 102, 106, 111, 116
dysfunctional, 111
dysmenorrhea, viii, 114
dysplasia, 44

E

economic, 104, 118
economic problem, 118
economic status, 104
eczema, 86, 87
edema, 28
education, 51, 71, 117
efficacy, 49, 62, 93, 95, 98, 109, 113
egg, 108
eicosanoids, 22
ejaculation, 108
elective abortion, 107
electronic, iv
electrostatic, iv
embolism, 11, 14, 21

embolus, 11, 19
embryo, 107
emotional, vii, 101, 102
encoding, 108
endocarditis, 61, 119
endocrinology, 120
endogenous, ix, 9, 26, 37, 42, 60, 86, 87
endometrial cancer, 37, 38, 51
endometrial carcinoma, 37
endometrial hyperplasia, 38, 51, 111
endometriosis, viii, 114
endometrium, vii, 38, 111, 112
endothelial cell, 30
endothelial cells, 30
endothelial dysfunction, 30
endothelium, 7, 13, 61
England, 22
Enhancement, xi, 12, 21
enlargement, 100
environment, ix, 18
enzyme, 62, 75
enzymes, 62
eosinophils, 30
epidemic, 56
epidemiologic studies, 6, 42, 109
epidemiological, 12, 36, 39, 46, 50, 52, 85
epidemiology, 41
epidermal, 43
epidermal growth factor, 43
epididymis, 108, 110
epilepsy, 61, 65, 66
epithelial cell, 34, 35, 49
epithelial cells, 34, 35, 49
epithelial ovarian cancer, 50, 51
epithelium, vii, 36
equilibrium, 86
erythema multiforme, 87, 90
erythema nodosum, 87, 90
erythematous, 60, 64, 66, 118, 121
esterase, 25
estimating, 47
estradiol, vii, 7, 9, 26, 34, 50, 82, 88, 90, 95, 112
estrogen, vii, ix, x, 1, 3, 5, 6, 7, 9, 10, 12, 13, 17, 20, 21, 22, 25, 26, 28, 35, 36, 38, 41, 43, 45, 46, 50, 51, 52, 54, 60, 61, 63, 72, 75, 77, 82, 84, 86, 87, 88, 89, 92, 110, 119
estrogen receptors, 35, 41, 77
estrogens, 7, 10, 13, 36, 39, 43, 45, 48, 51, 54, 60, 62, 76, 77, 86, 114
etiologic agent, 27
etiology, 30, 41, 90, 97
Europe, 56, 118
European, 44, 79
Europeans, 79
evidence, ix, 2, 5, 7, 12, 13, 14, 17, 18, 25, 34, 35, 36, 43, 44, 46, 48, 49, 50, 54, 80, 86, 91, 95, 103, 106, 109, 113
evolution, 56
examinations, 37
excretion, 12, 22, 63, 64, 65, 75
exogenous, 26, 37, 42, 46, 47, 49, 54, 59, 60, 64, 84, 86, 87
expert, iv, 119
exposure, 5, 43, 46, 47, 55, 56, 59, 84, 86, 88
expulsion, 107
extracellular, 91
eye, 27, 28, 29
eyes, 86

F

factor VII, 9, 11, 20
factor VIII, 20
failure, 62, 69, 81
familial, 37, 45, 54, 63, 70, 75
family, viii, ix, 7, 8, 10, 11, 12, 14, 18, 19, 37, 59, 73, 104, 105, 106, 110, 117
family history, ix, 10, 12, 14, 19, 59
family planning, viii, 73, 104, 105, 106, 117
fasting, 78
fat, 91
FDA, 100
fear, 92
fears, 113, 119
feet, 87
females, 55, 83, 87
fertility, ix, 62, 67, 74, 107, 108, 110, 112, 117, 120, 121
fertility regulation, 107, 112

Index

fertilization, 107
fever, 75, 87
fibrinogen, 1, 9
fibrinolysis, 11, 20
filtration, 22, 65, 67, 68
flare, 63
flora, 105, 107
flow, 96
fluctuations, 12, 96, 101
fluid, 13, 94
follicle, 99, 108
follicles, 99
follicle-stimulating hormone, 108
follicular, 99, 100, 101, 111
food, 26
food allergy, 26
Food and Drug Administration (FDA), 99
forgetting, 7
Fox, 86
fractures, 62
free radical, 13, 61
fungal, 105
fusion, 109

G

gamete, 108
gamma-aminobutyric acid, 101
gastrointestinal, 30, 60, 86
gastrointestinal tract, 30, 60
gene, 4, 6, 8, 16, 18, 19, 20, 25, 46, 64, 108
generation, vii, x, xi, 3, 6, 8, 10, 11, 12, 20, 21, 28, 60, 64, 68, 78, 92
genes, 37, 108, 109
genetic, 34, 35, 37, 49, 75, 114
genetics, 49, 85
genotype, 20
germline mutations, 37
gestation, 34
gestational diabetes, 78, 82
girls, ix, 40, 53, 86, 102
gland, 38
glucagon, 77
glucocorticoid receptor, 18
gluconeogenesis, 77

glucose, 23, 28, 77
glucose metabolism, 28, 77
glucose tolerance, 23, 77
glycogen, 44
glycosylated, 79
gonadotropin, 88, 108
Gram-negative, 106
Gram-positive, 106
groups, x, 78, 91, 96, 99, 100, 105, 109
growth, 34, 45, 46, 47, 50, 57, 58, 60, 66, 118
growth factor, 34, 50
growth factors, 35
guidance, 82, 114
guidelines, 66, 71
gynecologic cancer, 49, 51
gynecologist, 71, 113, 119
gynecologists, 40

H

HAART, 71
haemostasis, vii, 6, 15, 17
hair loss, 86
hands, 87
haplotype, 6, 17, 19
HDL, vii, 13, 78
headache, 28, 61, 84, 85, 91, 114
health, vii, x, xi, 36, 39, 51, 61, 72, 82, 84, 105, 109, 112, 115, 117, 118, 120
health care, xi, 72, 117
health education, 115
health effects, 36
heart, 5, 65, 70, 71, 118, 121
heart attack, 5
heart transplantation, 71
hemodynamic, 23
hemophilia, 19
hemorrhage, 27, 44
hemorrhagic stroke, 4
hemostasis, 7, 10, 18, 21, 80
hemostatic, ix, 9, 21, 82
hepatic failure, 27
hepatic transplant, 70
hepatitis, 45, 70
hepatitis B, 45

hepatocellular, 26, 44, 56, 57
hepatocellular carcinoma, 44, 56, 57
hepatocyte, 45
hereditary non-polyposis colorectal cancer, 37
herpes, 88
herpes simplex, 88
heterogeneous, 25, 29
hidradenitis suppurativa, 86
high risk, ix, 5, 8, 11, 19, 20, 37, 38, 39, 52, 60, 70, 81, 120
high school, 116
HIS, 85
Hispanic, 49
histological, 36
HIV, 40, 53, 61, 63, 66, 67, 71, 73, 74, 114, 117
HIV infection, 61, 71, 114
HIV/AIDS, 71
HIV-1, 63, 66, 72, 73
Holland, 53
homology, 109
homozygosity, 20, 64
hormonal therapy, 45
hormone, 3, 26, 36, 41, 46, 47, 54, 59, 62, 68, 72, 80, 83, 84, 88, 100, 102, 107, 108, 111
hormones, xi, 15, 22, 26, 29, 41, 43, 46, 47, 50, 52, 54, 57, 58, 59, 101, 105, 117
HSIL, 40, 72
human, 34, 39, 45, 47, 49, 50, 52, 53, 58, 59, 67, 73, 104, 107, 108, 109, 110, 120
human chorionic gonadotropin, 107, 108, 109
human immunodeficiency virus, 53, 67
human papilloma virus (HPV), 39, 52, 53, 72, 114, 117
humans, 45, 108, 111
hydroxylation, 39
hypercholesterolemia, 6
hypercoagulable, 11, 21
hyperhomocysteinemia, 5, 60
hyperinsulinism, 77
hyperlipidemia, 61, 81, 119
hyperplasia, 38, 44, 57, 58, 60, 64, 76, 77, 118, 119, 121
hyperplastic polyps, 54
hypersensitivity, 30, 86

hypertension, ix, 2, 3, 6, 12, 13, 14, 21, 22, 28, 61, 65, 66, 67, 68, 85
hypertensive, 12, 13, 23, 61
hypothalamic, 100, 112
hypothesis, 3, 46, 48
hysterectomy, 38, 41, 52

I

iatrogenic, 25, 29
id, 101
identification, 120, 121
identity, 109
idiopathic, xii, 10, 21, 25
idiosyncratic, 103
IgE, 30
IGF, 42
IGF-I, 42
imbalances, 34
immune response, 108
immune system, 31, 108
immunity, 31
immunization, 107, 109, 110
immunodeficiency, 40
immunogenicity, 109
immunological, 107
immunosuppression, 40
immunosuppressive, 30, 67, 70, 105
immunosuppressive agent, 70, 105
immunosuppressive drugs, 67
implants, 34, 61, 95, 97, 114, 119
in situ, 39, 41
in vitro, 30, 35, 47, 108
incidence, vii, 1, 3, 4, 15, 19, 27, 28, 36, 39, 44, 47, 51, 55, 59, 62, 67, 69, 91, 93, 96, 99, 119
income, 117
index case, 29
India, 28
Indian, 26, 28, 97
indication, 88, 112
indicators, 104
induction, 62
industrialized countries, 92, 102
infarction, 2, 5, 7, 13, 15, 16, 84, 85

infection, 4, 40, 53, 69, 70, 72
infections, 40, 52, 68, 73, 105
infectious, 61, 119
infertile, 109
infertility, 41, 102, 109
inflammation, 6, 17, 30
ingestion, 42
inherited, 2, 4, 8, 18, 19, 25, 26, 49, 51, 61
inhibition, 43, 109
inhibitor, 25, 71, 83, 100, 108, 109, 110
inhibitory, 35, 111
inhibitory effect, 35, 111
initiation, 79, 88
injection, 114
injections, 62, 119
injury, iv
insertion, 39, 40, 115, 117
insight, 66
insulin, xii, 42, 44, 77, 82
insulin dependent diabetes, 44, 78, 82
insulin resistance, 77, 82
insulin sensitivity, 79
insulin-like growth factor, 42
integration, 81, 101
intensity, 84
interaction, 3, 8, 18, 104, 108, 111
interleukin, 40, 72
interleukin-1, 40
international, vii, xi, 15, 34, 48, 120
International Agency for Research on Cancer, (IARC), 39, 45, 53
interrelations, 28
interval, 84, 85
intervention, 73, 116
intracerebral, 4
intracranial, 59
intramuscular, 72, 87, 88
intramuscular injection, 88
intraocular, 28
intraocular pressure, 28
intraperitoneal, 27, 44
intrauterine contraceptive device, 67, 106
intrinsic, 8, 107
invasive, 39, 52, 117
invasive cancer, 52

irrational anxieties, vii
irritability, 102
IRS, 42
ischemic, 4, 13, 16, 17
ischemic stroke, 4, 13, 16, 17
Italy, 1, 33, 55, 59, 106

J

JAMA, 49, 90, 99
jaundice, 75
Jordan, 14
Jun, 49, 51, 73

K

kidney, 13, 22, 61, 65, 67, 68, 69
kidney failure, 13, 22, 61, 65
kidney transplant, 69
kidney transplantation, 69
kidneys, 27, 30, 60

L

laceration, 87
lactation, 36, 47
language, 113
latency, 47
Latin America, 119
Latino, 82
Latino women, 82
laws, 119
LDL, 13, 78
lead, vii, ix, 7, 10, 27, 30, 60, 63, 77, 92, 95, 114, 119
lens, 28
lesions, 27, 30, 40, 41, 53, 87, 89
libido, 103, 104
life cycle, 103
lifestyle, x, 42, 114
life-threatening, 11, 30, 85, 86
lifetime, 37, 106
ligands, 110
limitations, 4

linear, 46
links, 46
lipid, vii, 10, 13, 23, 28, 61, 70, 77, 82, 83
lipid metabolism, 23, 70, 77, 82, 83
lipid profile, 13, 79
lipids, 78, 82
lipoprotein, 82, 83
lipoproteins, viii, 80
literature, 42, 47, 90
liver, vii, 27, 44, 56, 57, 58, 60, 63, 64, 66, 68, 69, 70, 75, 77, 83
liver disease, 60, 64, 66, 69, 75
liver failure, 27
liver function tests, 70
liver transplant, 69, 70
liver transplantation, 69, 70
LNG, 9, 10, 11, 12, 35, 38, 78, 87, 91, 95, 104
locus, 109
London, 63, 120
long period, 44
longitudinal study, 82
long-term, viii, 34, 36, 39, 42, 45, 56, 57, 68, 69, 70, 72, 80, 83, 89, 94, 113, 120
losses, 80
LSIL, 40, 72
lungs, 27
lupus, 60, 61, 64, 66, 86, 118, 121
lupus erythematosus, 86
luteinizing hormone, 109
lymph, 27
lymph node, 27
lymphocyte, 30, 63, 72
lymphocytes, 30

M

M.O., 64
magnetic, iv
malaise, 87
Malaysia, 29
malignant, 13, 33, 34, 44, 46, 55, 56, 57, 61, 87
malignant melanoma, 44, 55, 56, 87
management, ix, x, 7, 49, 65, 86, 97, 100, 115
market, viii

mass media, vii
mastectomy, 35
maternal, 120
maturation, 34, 108, 111
measurement, 25, 102
measures, 35, 92
mechanical, iv
media, vii
median, 41
medication, 29, 44
medications, 4, 93, 98
melanoma, 43, 55, 56
men, 1, 42, 46, 47, 74, 101, 109, 117, 120
menarche, 34, 46, 47
meningioma, 48, 59
menopausal, viii, xi, 7, 10, 29, 41, 47
menopause, ix, 30, 41, 47, 65, 101
menstrual, vii, ix, 39, 41, 67, 69, 87, 91, 94, 97, 104, 111, 114, 119
menstrual cycle, ix, 67, 68, 87, 96, 111, 114, 119
menstrual irregularity, 114
menstruation, viii, 35, 88, 92, 112, 113, 116
meta-analysis, xi, 6, 14, 15, 17
metabolic, 61, 62, 71, 80, 82, 83, 119
metabolism, viii, 62, 79, 82, 83
metabolite, viii
mice, 108
microflora, 62
middle class, 92
migraine, 3, 5, 7, 15, 17, 28, 61, 65, 84, 85
migraine headache, 61, 84
migraine with aura, 5, 7, 84
migraine without aura, 84
migraines, 28
mild hypertensive, 22
mimicking, 89
minority, 46
miscarriage, 79, 101
misconceptions, 29
mitosis, 34
mitotic, 35, 111
modulation, 101, 113
molecular biology, 120
molecules, 108, 110, 121

monkeys, 108, 112
monotherapy, 65
mood, 61, 101, 103, 105
mood change, 101, 103
mood disorder, 61, 101, 103
mortality, 6, 44, 47, 59, 71, 120
mouse, 109
MPA, 34, 40, 47, 102
mucosa, 42, 86
multiple sclerosis, 4
multivariate, 42, 72
muscle, 60
muscle strength, 60
muscles, 30, 60
mutation, viii, xi, 2, 4, 8, 10, 11, 12, 19, 20, 21, 31, 34, 35, 37, 48, 60, 64, 114
mutations, 8, 25, 35, 37, 46, 50, 54
myocardial infarction, xii, 1, 5, 7, 13, 14, 15, 17, 61, 81

N

N-acety, 54
natural, 19, 85, 88, 104, 105
nausea, 91
necrosis, 26, 27, 31, 32
necrotizing glomerulonephritis, 30
necrotizing systemic vasculitis, 30
necrotizing vasculitis, 30, 60
negative mood, 102, 104
neoplasia, 55
neoplasm, 41
neoplasms, x
neoplastic, 4, 8, 33, 34, 46, 119
neoplastic diseases, 8
nephritis, 63, 119
nephropathy, 66, 67, 69, 121
nephrotic syndrome, 5, 60
nephrotoxicity, 67
nerve, 46
nerves, 30, 60
neurofibroma, 46
neuropathy, 28
New York, iii, iv, 54, 81
Newton, 103

NHC, 78
Nigeria, 117
nodules, 58, 64, 87, 118, 121
non-immunological, 68
non-nucleoside reverse transcriptase inhibitors, 63
non-smokers, 2
normal, 8, 25, 34, 67, 69, 79, 95
nucleus, 70
nulliparous, 34, 43, 46

O

Obese, 80
obesity, ix, 12, 42, 61, 85
observations, 36, 45, 79, 112
obstruction, 25
occlusion, 4, 6, 18, 27, 28
occupational, 58
OCs, 2, 29, 34, 42, 106
odds ratio, 2, 3, 4, 40, 46, 102, 106
ODN, 110
oedema, 25, 26, 91
oestrogen, 18, 21, 26, 38, 85
office-based, 83
Oncology, 33, 55
oocyte, 107
oocytes, 108
oophorectomy, 41, 47, 50, 88
ophthalmic, 28, 29
oral, vii, xi, xii, 2, 4, 6, 7, 11, 12, 13, 14, 15, 16, 17, 19, 20, 21, 22, 23, 25, 26, 27, 28, 29, 30, 32, 34, 35, 36, 37, 39, 41, 43, 44, 46, 48, 50, 51, 52, 53, 54, 55, 56, 57, 58, 60, 63, 64, 65, 66, 68, 70, 72, 76, 77, 82, 83, 84, 87, 88, 89, 90, 92, 93, 94, 95, 97, 98, 100, 101, 103, 104, 105, 106, 107, 115, 116, 117, 118, 119, 121
oral cavity, 87
oral contraceptives, vii, xi, xii, 4, 6, 7, 11, 12, 13, 14, 15, 16, 17, 19, 20, 21, 22, 23, 25, 26, 27, 28, 29, 31, 34, 35, 36, 37, 39, 41, 43, 44, 48, 50, 51, 52, 53, 54, 55, 56, 57, 58, 60, 63, 64, 65, 66, 76, 77, 82, 83, 84,

87, 88, 90, 92, 93, 95, 97, 98, 101, 104, 105, 106, 107, 115, 116, 117, 118, 119, 121
organ, 30, 69
organism, 105
osteoporosis, 62
ovarian, 34, 35, 36, 38, 49, 50, 51, 99, 100, 101, 108, 120
ovarian cancer, 35, 36, 38, 49, 50, 51
ovarian cancers, 35, 36, 38, 50
ovarian cysts, 99, 100, 101
ovaries, 47
ovary, 45
overpopulation, 118
overweight, 8, 80
oviduct, 111
ovulation, vii, ix, 62, 83, 100, 111
ovum, 107

P

p53, 54
pain, 25, 26, 60, 75
pancreas, 77
pancreatic, 46, 58, 59
pancreatic cancer, 46, 58, 59
panic attack, 102
panic disorder, 103
paradox, 41
parathyroid, 27
parathyroid glands, 27
parenchyma, 27
parenthood, 68
Paris, x, 18, 20, 29, 53, 64, 66, 71, 76, 81, 83, 90
partial thromboplastin time, 9
partnerships, ix, 114
pathogenesis, 4, 18, 27, 49, 52, 56, 117
pathogenic, 37
pathology, 5, 10, 17
patients, xi, 3, 19, 25, 30, 31, 35, 44, 46, 57, 58, 60, 61, 63, 65, 66, 67, 70, 71, 84, 106, 116, 118, 119, 121
pearls, 31
peptide, 77, 108
periodic, 111

peripheral arterial disease, 6, 17
peripheral nerve, 45
permeability, 28
permit, 28, 34, 115
personal, vii, 14, 59, 114
pH, 86
phagocytic, 27
pharmaceutical, vii, 86
pharmaceutical companies, vii
pharmacokinetics, 67
pharmacological, 119
phospholipids, 79
phosphorylation, 47, 59
photosensitivity, 86
physicians, 94
physiology, 11
pilot study, 84, 85, 98
pituitary, 100, 111
placebo, 42, 85, 91, 93
placental, 107
planning, 81
plaques, 87
plasma, 9, 23, 77
plasma levels, 23
platelet, 9, 13, 61
platelet count, 9
play, vii, ix, 13, 25, 46, 47
political, 120
Polyarteritis nodosa, 30, 31, 60, 64
polycystic ovary syndrome, 58
polymorphism, 6
polymorphisms, 54
polyp, 42, 54
polyps, 41, 54
poor, vii, ix, 80, 102, 114
POPs, 62
population, 3, 8, 19, 34, 44, 46, 59, 64, 76, 85, 91, 104, 105, 107, 109, 118, 120
population growth, 107
porphyria, 59, 64, 76, 86, 89
portal hypertension, 27
portal vein, 77
positive mood, 102
postmenopausal, 38, 46, 47
postmenopausal women, 46, 47

Index

postpartum, 78, 117
precancer, 40
prednisone, 70
pre-eclampsia, 2
pre-existing, 5, 13, 34, 61, 82
preference, 115
pregnancy, viii, ix, xi, 2, 7, 12, 16, 26, 29, 34, 36, 43, 44, 46, 67, 68, 69, 70, 72, 75, 78, 84, 86, 92, 96, 98, 101, 105, 107, 108, 111, 113, 115, 116, 117, 119, 120
pregnant, 43, 72, 113
premenopausal, 46
premenstrual dysphoric disorder, 101
preparation, iv, 3, 5, 80, 95
pressure, 3, 12, 13, 61, 68
prevention, 17, 37, 49, 53, 73, 80, 120
preventive, xi, 5, 35, 60, 84, 117
procedures, 8
procoagulant, 1, 11, 18
production, 13, 61, 87, 100, 108
progesterone, 3, 5, 25, 34, 36, 38, 42, 43, 46, 50, 52, 58, 61, 63, 72, 87, 88, 89, 90, 100, 110, 112, 113, 120, 121
progestins, vii, ix, 5, 7, 8, 10, 11, 12, 13, 18, 28, 36, 43, 50, 60, 68, 77, 82, 92, 104, 111, 113
prognosis, 27
progressive, 30, 40, 60, 67, 70, 99
proliferation, 35, 45, 49, 58, 112
promote, 6, 43, 63, 72, 73, 116
promoter, 39
property, iv, 86
prophylactic, 35, 50
prophylaxis, 70
proposition, 108
proptosis, 28
prostaglandin, 42
prostaglandins, 111
prostate, 108
prostate specific antigen, 108
protease inhibitors, 63, 108, 110
protection, 36, 37, 41, 62, 72, 108
protein, xi, 4, 8, 12, 16, 19, 20, 60, 64, 108, 109, 114
proteinase, 30

proteins, 108, 110, 121
prothrombin, 2, 4, 8, 19
proto-oncogene, 43
pruritus, 75, 86, 87
psyche, 102
psychological, vii, 101, 103, 105
puberty, 34, 46
public, 36, 39, 104, 107
public health, 107
pulmonary embolism, xii, 1, 11, 61
pulmonary hypertension, 61, 119
pyoderma gangrenosum, 32

Q

quality of life, x, 67, 97, 120

R

range, 86
rash, 75
reactivity, 13, 61
reality, vii
recall, 49
receptor agonist, 101
receptors, 7, 9, 11, 42, 45, 63, 89, 110
recurrence, 106
reduction, vii, 9, 10, 28, 36, 41, 46, 60, 71, 75, 77, 82, 92, 96, 99, 101, 107
Registry, 55
regression, 27, 42, 54, 56
regular, 111, 114, 115
regulation, 82, 120
relationship, vii, 5, 12, 22, 28, 39, 41, 49, 69, 72, 85, 88, 92, 104, 105, 106
relationships, 87, 101
relevance, 120
religious, 119
remission, 38, 60, 100
renal, 30, 61, 63, 67, 68, 71
renal disease, 63
renin, 13
repair, 6, 37
replication, 43

reproduction, 72, 120
reproductive age, 60, 99
reproductive organs, 48
research, vii, 5, 6, 47, 107, 120
researchers, 34, 41, 106, 108
resistance, 9, 12, 20, 60, 64, 78
resolution, 28, 87, 99
respiratory, 30
responsiveness, ix
restoration, 69
retention, 13, 92
retina, 28
retinopathy, 28
returns, 13, 61
Reynolds, 66
rheumatic, 66
rheumatic diseases, 66
rheumatoid arthritis, 30
rhythm, 61, 119
rings, 12, 119
risk, viii, ix, x, xi, 1, 3, 4, 6, 7, 10, 11, 12, 13, 14, 15, 16, 17, 18, 19, 20, 21, 22, 23, 27, 28, 30, 33, 34, 36, 37, 39, 41, 43, 44, 46, 47, 48, 49, 50, 51, 52, 53, 54, 55, 56, 57, 58, 59, 60, 63, 65, 67, 69, 70, 72, 73, 77, 84, 92, 96, 100, 101, 106, 108, 111, 114, 119
risk assessment, 51, 56
risk factors, 2, 3, 4, 6, 7, 13, 14, 17, 18, 20, 27, 41, 54, 55, 68, 77, 84, 106
risks, vii, x, 2, 3, 8, 14, 40, 42, 47, 53, 65, 70, 85, 115
RNA, 63
rosacea, 87, 89

S

safety, viii, ix, 7, 10, 62, 83, 98, 99, 107, 108, 119
salpingo-oophorectomy, 35
salt, 23
Sao Paulo, 57
Sartorius, 105
satisfaction, x, 69, 93, 97, 103, 105
Schiff, 56
Schmid, 58
Schwann cells, 46, 58
scientific, vii
sclerosis, 28
Seattle, 54
second generation, 3, 6, 11
secretion, 77
seizure, 4, 62
seizures, 60
Self, 114, 116
semen, 109
sensitivity, 9, 101, 104, 111
sequelae, 75
sequencing, 110
serine, 108
serum, 3, 37, 68, 78, 88, 109
services, iv, viii
severity, 31, 64, 84, 89
sex, 7, 9, 36, 45, 57, 62, 64, 68, 101, 104, 108, 116
sex hormones, 36, 45, 64
sex steroid, 45, 57, 108
sexual behavio(u)r, viii, 104, 106, 114
sexual intercourse, viii, 39, 114
sexuality, 67, 103, 105
sexually transmitted disease, 72, 73, 114, 120
sexually transmitted diseases, 72, 73, 114
shock, 27
short period, 114
Short-term, 12
side effects, 61, 93, 97, 98, 105, 113, 119
signaling, 43
signs, 28
similarity, 78
Singapore, 58, 76, 121
sinus, 5, 15, 16, 60, 64
skin, 25, 26, 29, 31, 43, 54, 55, 56, 60, 86, 87, 88
skin cancer, 43, 54
SLE, 62, 66, 119
smoke, 2, 5, 6, 13, 81, 85
smokers, x, 3
smoking, 2, 3, 6, 15, 28, 41, 54
smoking cessation, 6
smooth muscle, 7, 9, 11

smooth muscle cells, 7, 9
social, ix, 101, 102, 103, 114, 118
social status, 101
socialization, 101
sodium, 13
South Africa, 63, 89
Southeast Asia, 119
species, 105, 109, 111
specific knowledge, x
specificity, 30
sperm, 107, 110
sperm function, 109
spleen, 27
spontaneous abortion, 34
sporadic, ix, 3, 5, 25, 28, 35, 60, 102
squamous cell, 40
stages, 40, 41
sterile, 109
sterilization, 70, 104, 105
steroid, viii, xii, 15, 20, 30, 43, 50, 52, 56, 57, 62, 99, 112, 117
steroid hormone, 52, 117
steroids, vii, 3, 7, 9, 18, 45, 63, 81, 101, 104, 108, 119
STI, 72
stimulus, 88
storage, 44
strategies, 112, 120
stratification, 16
stress, 101
stroke, 3, 4, 7, 13, 15, 16, 17, 61, 84, 85
stroma, 38
stromal, 38
stromal cells, 39
students, 116
subdural hematoma, 4
subgroups, 85
sub-Saharan Africa, 119
substances, 75
substitution, 1, 37
success rate, 114
suffering, x, 61, 64, 84
sugar, 80
sulfonamides, 62
Sun, 16

sunlight, 86
supplements, 85
suppression, 22, 113
surgeries, 35
surgery, 35, 37
surgical, 8, 67, 70
surveillance, 35, 37, 40, 45
survival, 67, 70
survivors, 69
susceptibility, 37, 42, 64, 89
susceptibility genes, 37
sustainability, 83
Sweden, 64
switching, x
Switzerland, 32, 99
sympathetic, 13, 61
symptoms, viii, 25, 28, 30, 35, 91, 94, 101, 105
syndrome, 30, 31, 32, 37, 45, 50, 61, 63, 76, 86, 89, 119
synthetic, vii, 3, 10, 50, 63, 77, 87, 109
systematic, 14, 15, 52
systematic review, 14, 15, 52
systemic lupus erythematosus, 59, 66, 86, 89
systems, 75, 96, 98, 101, 119
systolic pressure, 13

T

tamoxifen, 35, 88
target organs, vii
targets, 121
T-cell, 40
technology, 120
teenagers, viii, 114
teens, 79
telangiectasia, 18
tension, 92
testis, 108, 110
testosterone, ix, 35, 50, 104
testosterone levels, 104
Thai, 19, 53, 93, 98, 100
Thailand, 98
theory, 73, 116

therapy, viii, 18, 26, 29, 36, 38, 41, 45, 46, 54, 56, 60, 62, 67, 70, 80, 84, 86, 90, 100, 102, 105
Thomson, 49
threatening, 25, 31, 89
threshold, 108
thrombin, 7, 9, 11, 18
thromboembolic, x, 3, 20, 21, 61, 119
thromboembolism, ix, xi, xii, 4, 7, 11, 15, 17, 18, 19, 20, 21
thrombophlebitis, 21, 68, 87, 89
thrombosis, xi, xii, 2, 5, 6, 9, 10, 11, 12, 14, 15, 16, 17, 18, 19, 20, 21, 28, 29, 45, 58, 60, 64, 118, 119, 121
thrombotic, 7, 9, 11, 14, 60, 84
thyroid, 47, 59, 83
thyroid cancer, 47, 59
time, viii, 9, 34, 36, 38, 45, 67, 70, 80, 84, 92, 96, 101, 109, 112, 114, 119
timing, 101
TNF, 30
TNF-alpha, 30
tobacco, 85
tolerance, 77, 93, 94
total cholesterol, 78
toxicity, 7, 10, 29
training, 114
traits, 55
transcription, 39
transdermal patch, viii, 5, 21, 114
transformation, 38, 44, 46, 57
transgenic, 120
transition, xi
transmission, 71, 73
transnational, 2
transplant, 67, 68, 69, 70, 71, 115, 118
transplant recipients, 68, 71, 118
transplantation, 67, 68, 69
trend, 42, 46, 59, 72, 80, 115
trial, 42, 67, 73, 74, 83, 88, 93, 97, 103, 108
triglyceride, 78
triglycerides, 78
tubal ligation, 36
tumor, 43, 45, 46, 48, 56, 57, 63
tumor growth, 63

tumors, 33, 35, 36, 44, 46, 56
type 1 diabetes, 81, 83, 84, 118
type 2 diabetes, 81
type 2 diabetes mellitus, 81

U

UAE, 12
ulceration, 87, 89
ultrasonography, 38, 45
Ultraviolet (UV), 43, 55
unilateral, 28
United States, x, 21, 33, 54, 59, 61, 92, 116, 120
urban, 117
urinary, 12, 22, 64, 65
urine, 60
urticaria, 25, 30, 86, 87, 89
users, x, 1, 3, 4, 7, 8, 10, 12, 15, 16, 17, 20, 22, 27, 33, 35, 36, 38, 39, 41, 44, 47, 51, 60, 63, 72, 76, 78, 91, 94, 97, 98, 99, 101, 103, 113
uterus, 113
UV exposure, 43

V

Vaccination, 109
vaccine, 107
vaccines, 108, 109, 120
vagina, 87, 111
vaginal, 5, 12, 37, 80, 83, 90, 91, 93, 95, 97, 102, 104, 105, 107, 114
vaginitis, 106
values, 78
variable, 28, 29, 96, 109, 110
variables, 6, 21, 82, 106
variation, 4, 12, 16, 92, 94
vascular, viii, 3, 7, 8, 10, 11, 13, 17, 18, 22, 27, 28, 29, 60, 61, 62, 80, 86, 119
vascular disease, 17, 22
vascular diseases, 17
vascular occlusion, 29
vasculitis, 29, 31, 90

Index

vein, xi, 5, 7, 9, 10, 11, 12, 19, 21, 28, 29, 45, 60, 61, 64, 119
ventricular, 61, 119
venules, 29
vessels, 30
viral, 69
viral hepatitis, 69
virus, 72, 73
viruses, 45
vision, 27, 28
visual, 5, 17, 28
vitamin C, 61
vitamin D, 62
vomiting, 60, 75
vulnerability, 101

W

Washington, 54, 59
water, 91
Watson, 50
Wegener's granulomatosis, 30, 31, 32
weight changes, 91
weight control, 81
weight gain, viii, 91
weight loss, 75
weight status, 94
well-being, 94, 104, 105
whey, 109
white women, 48, 49
withdrawal, 12, 44, 56, 84, 95, 111
Wnt signaling, 57
World Health Organisation (WHO), 15, 20, 40, 71, 108

Y

yeast, 106
young women, ix, 4, 6, 8, 13, 14, 15, 17, 28, 34, 40, 44, 45, 49, 56, 60, 71, 81, 91, 97, 102, 120, 121

Z

zygote, 107